YOUR CHILD'S ASTHMA

A Guide for Parents

YOUR CHILD'S ASTHMA

A Guide for Parents

John Hunt, MD, FAAAAI

Pediatrician,
Pediatric Pulmonologist,
Pediatric Allergist/Immunologist

Illustrations by Lauren Rakes

Printed in the United States of America.

ISBN: 978-09-8593-321-0 (print)

ISBN: 978-09-8593-322-7 (ebook)

Acknowledgments and Dedication

I gratefully acknowledge the doctors and nurses who mentored me in all things asthma, but particularly: Ben Gaston, MD; Thomas A.E. Platts-Mills, FRS, MD, PhD; Peter Heymann, MD; Jackie Brown, RN; and Deb Murphy, RN. Much thanks to I. Harry David, Nathalie Marcus, and B.K. Marcus from Invisible Order.

This book is dedicated to Professor Freddy Hargreave, MD, MB, FRCPC, FRCP—a humble, brilliant, and perfectly kind human being—who had asthma figured out better than anyone, and who we all so sorely miss.

Contents

Foreword

I t is not often that one gets to read a handbook for patients written by a physician without the slightest tone of condescendence, particularly when the book is directed at the parents of children with chronic disease. This remarkable book is written by an exceptional down-to-earth physician and educator who has years of experience in clinical medicine and an extraordinary sense of humility and the need to give back to his community.

Dr. Hunt wrote *Your Child's Asthma* respectful of the intelligence of parents. He recognizes that not only are parents wise about their children, but, with a little effort, parents can become just as wise about asthma.

He provides experienced insight into the mechanisms of asthma and presents a method of determining treatments based on the underlying physiological problems that are found to be relevant in each individual child. He does not condone cookbook medicine, nor promote the blind following of treatment guidelines written by scientists who have never met your child.

Dr. Hunt explains the scientific underpinnings of all symptoms that children may experience and then provides clear lucid explanations for the common and not so common factors that are likely to trigger an asthma attack in children. This holistic approach is a reflection of his academic career and his research inquisitiveness that are complemented by his extraordinary qualities as a caring physician.

Dr. Hunt dedicates this book to Professor Freddy Hargreave, and that is appropriate indeed. Over an illustrious career spanning 40 years,

Professor Hargreave applied research methods to improve the care that he provided to his patients at McMaster University. He pioneered the use of measurements of airway hyperresponsiveness and airway inflammation to diagnose and to guide therapy for various airway diseases such as those that cause asthma.

Dr. Hunt has faithfully applied Professor Hargreave's principles in asserting the importance of accurately diagnosing patients, both in his clinical practice and in this handbook. By its creative and informative illustrations, and scientific yet practical approach and narrative, this book is unique and will serve as a valuable resource for young patients and their parents and caregivers.

Parameswaran Nair, MD, PhD, FRCP, FRCPC
Canada Research Chair in Airway Inflammometry
Professor of Medicine, McMaster University
Adjunct Professor of Medicine, McGill University
Staff Respirologist, St. Joseph's Healthcare Hamilton,
   Ontario, Canada
April 2015

Introduction

This book is focused on helping you improve *your* child's asthma. Your child's asthma may be similar to or entirely different from the asthma that other children have. Different forms of asthma need very different treatments. This book will help you determine what type (*or types*) of asthma *your* child has, so that the right course of action can be chosen to combat it.

Some of the information in this book may help you to understand your child's *past* asthma when he was younger. Some of the information may help you anticipate your child's *future* with asthma. Much is focused on the *now*. The information in this book may even help you and your child's doctor recognize a diagnosis for your child's asthma that neither of you had considered. This book is designed to help you be the best partner to your child's doctor in optimally managing your child's asthma.

It is fair for you to want to know about the doctor who wrote this book.

I was fortunate to be trained in both of the two pediatric subspecialty fields that separately provide care to children who have asthma. I thus became both a pediatric pulmonologist (lung physician) and an allergist/immunologist. My mentors are brilliant and wonderful physicians who have generously shared their wisdom with me. I had the honor of working with some of the best minds in asthma when I was the chairman of the Asthma Diagnosis and Pharmacotherapeutics Committee of the American Academy of Allergy, Asthma, and Immunology. My academic career took me through a position as a tenured associate professor

3

of pediatric respiratory medicine at the University of Virginia—a highly respected center of asthma research and clinical practice. During that time I was an author of one of the influential European pediatric asthma guidelines.

Although I have lived asthma *professionally* for more than two decades, what may be more important is that I have lived it *personally* as well.

I had severe asthma as a child myself. My children have asthma now. So, in that way, you and I are floating in the same boat.

I hope to be an advisor to you, a source of information, and a provider of reassurance. I hope to assist in improving your child's (and your) quality of life, and in decreasing unnecessary worry. It is my desire to empower you. A key component of empowerment is knowledge.

This book is about diagnosing, understanding, and treating the *individual* child with asthma—*your* child with asthma. I will repeat over and over again the core concept that *your child is an individual*. Other concepts are also occasionally repeated in two or more locations in the book. This repetition serves to incorporate the concepts into the various different contexts that you discover may be relevant to your child's asthma.

I wrote this book from the perspective of an allopath, which is the type of doctor I am. MD's are allopaths. I am not a naturopath, nor a nutritionist, nor a homeopath, nor any other alternative or complementary practitioner. All of these other professions have much to offer. I urge you to hear the suggestions of other professionals as well as my thoughts, and determine for yourself and your child what combination of the various medical philosophies seems most true and makes the most sense to you. I am confident that this book you are reading now will provide you critical knowledge to help you put other professionals' suggestions, and the suggestions of your doctor, your grandmother, your mother-in-law, and your neighbor's cousin's girlfriend, all into context.

It is also important to note that this book is not based on published *asthma guidelines* in the United States. Guidelines in medicine are compilations crafted by experts in which data are considered and treatment methods developed for optimization of average population outcomes. This book, however, is focused on helping *you* figure out what is going on with *your child,* not the average child. Unlike the experts who wrote the guidelines, you know *your child.* And that is so incredibly important!

As a result of years of consideration, I have learned to define asthma a bit differently than the writers of the US guidelines have recently defined it. My preferred definition of asthma eliminates some of the confusion that currently exists in the field of asthma.

I am a pediatrician. Part of my brain (perhaps an insufficient part) maintains a childlike view of the world, along with a willingness to use vocabulary that is perfectly descriptive yet entirely nonmedical. I will, without fear or hesitation, use the terms "booger" and "snot" (and whatever other phrases make sense at a given moment), and I may even define them. If the use of such language offends, I submit to you my sincere apologies.

I invite you to visit my website www.childasthmaguide.com for helpful information, updates, hints, reassurance, suggestions, and to learn about new discoveries.

Are you ready? Let's go!

CHAPTER 1

Asthma Is Not a Diagnosis

Your car develops a rattle.
You are worried about the rattle and want to know what is causing it.
You take your car to your mechanic.
Your mechanic listens to what you say and hears your car's rattle.
Your mechanic then tells you that the trouble with your car is a "rattle."
He charges you $100.
You get a new mechanic.

Rattle is not a diagnosis. It is a symptom. Something is causing your car to rattle and that something needs to be identified (diagnosed) in order to fix it.

Asthma is no more of a diagnosis than "rattle" is a diagnosis. I would ask that you allow me to repeat that concept. *Asthma is* not *a diagnosis*.

The nearly universal mistake that is made in dealing with asthma is considering asthma to be a diagnosis. Your recognition that "asthma" is *not* a diagnosis is the key first step in improving how you can deal with your child's asthma.

To help clarify, "the common cold" is a diagnosis. "Bacterial pneumonia" is a diagnosis. But in contrast, "cough" is *not* a diagnosis. Lots of different diseases can cause cough. We want to seek what causes the cough. And the cause we find for the cough is the *diagnosis*. And just like cough, "asthma" is not a diagnosis.

Asthma is a reason to go looking for a cause *for the asthma. Whatever is causing the asthma is the real "diagnosis."*

If asthma is not a diagnosis, what is it?

Asthma is a *physiologic disturbance.*

With asthma, something isn't working correctly in your child's windpipes, and this leads to a *symptom complex* that people call *asthma.* I'll discuss this more in the next chapter. The physiologic disturbance that leads to the symptoms people call *asthma* can result from very different pathologic processes (meaning very different diagnoses—indeed *entirely different diseases*). And these diseases, although they cause nearly identical symptoms, often require *entirely different therapies.*

The common *symptoms* found in a child with *asthma* are various combinations of

- Wheezing
- Coughing
- Shortness of breath
- Gurgling in the chest from accumulation of airway mucus
- Coughing up of mucus
- Anxiety/fear (from being short of breath)
- Inability to exercise during episodes
- Sometimes vomiting with coughing
- Tickling in the airway, under the chin, or in the front of the neck

Wheezing is the whistling of airflow through airways that are narrowed from any cause. *Coughing* results from the tickling of nerves in the airway, from any cause. *Shortness of breath* is known in the medical dictionary as *dyspnea,* and occurs in association with any disorder that causes insufficient oxygen and carbon dioxide exchange. *Mucus* production in the airways is a response to many lung conditions and injuries and infections. I can keep going, but the point is that the symptoms that occur in children with asthma overlap with the symptoms of all sorts of lung diseases.

If your child has these sorts of symptoms, it may be asthma (or may not be), and in any event, we want to seek what underlies the symptoms. What is the diagnosis?

There was once a television commercial that starred a guy who was dressed as a doctor stating in a deep voice with a serious tone, "I would like to talk to you for a moment about ... *diarrhea*." That ad made me cringe. So it is with some trepidation that I am about to engage in a brief deviation from asthma in order to talk to you for a moment about ... umm ... diarrhea. But just for a moment, I promise.

Here is a list of *causes* of diarrhea:

- Bacteria
- Viruses
- Parasites
- Anatomic abnormalities of the gut
- Autoimmune disorders
- Toxins
- Lactose intolerance
- Gluten enteropathy
- Ingestion of food that the gut is not tolerant of
- Stress/anxiety
- Allergies to ingested foods (allergies are a special type of intolerance)
- Tumors or masses in the gut

These are all radically different causes for diarrhea. Identifying the cause of the diarrhea from the above list takes you pretty close to a *diagnosis* for what is causing a given person's "diarrhea." Of course if you want to treat the diarrhea, you will treat it with one of many very different therapies that targets the underlying diagnosis.

I will now ask a silly question with an obvious answer:

Given that there are multiple different causes of diarrhea, would you want the doctor to diagnose your child with "diarrhea," and then *not* look for the cause? Should the doctor just treat your child with a cocktail of drugs for "diarrhea" according to a preset guideline written by experts who have never seen your child, never talked to you, never examined your child's stool under a microscope, and *never determined or even attempted to guess at the underlying diagnosis*? Do you want your child treated as a statistic as if every child with diarrhea has the same disease?

Of course not.

Because without a diagnosis, your child may be given the wrong therapy and be sicker than he needs to be, and for longer than he needs to be. Optimally, you would want your doctor to figure out what specifically is wrong with your child that has caused the diarrhea.

To the extent reasonable and possible, physicians should try to diagnose the cause of the symptom first and then treat the specific cause with therapies that have been proven to work for that cause. Now, a complete diagnosis is not always possible to obtain, nor is it always immediately certain (in fact, the passage of time is a great diagnostic ally). But it sure is helpful to have the true diagnosis when it is possible or reasonable to find it. When the choice of therapy depends so much on the cause of the problem (as is the case in diarrhea and asthma), trying to identify a specific diagnosis simply makes sense.

Now, as this is a book about asthma, let's get back to asthma. Like diarrhea, asthma is caused by all sorts of very different processes. Here is an incomplete list of those causes. You will see parallels to diarrhea! Note that this list of causes of asthma is not at all in order of frequency.

- Bacteria
- Viruses
- Parasites
- Anatomic abnormalities of the airways
- Autoimmune disorders
- Immunologic disturbances
- Toxins
- Aspiration of stomach or mouth contents into lung
- Food intolerances
- Stress/anxiety
- Allergies to stuff inhaled into the lung
- Tumors or masses in the lung
- Foreign objects inhaled into the airway

There are all these different causes for asthma—all these *very different potential diagnoses* for the diseases that cause someone to have asthma. Clearly, the optimal *treatments* for asthma are also going to be very different, and depend on the underlying diagnosis (in addition to the special characteristics of each child).

In the US, we all know that our medical system is a mess. And oh, what a mess! In this book, I am not going to discuss this mess, nor how to fix it, other than to reiterate that diagnosis is very important in selecting treatment, and if people in power misdiagnose the reason for the health-system mess, they will keep prescribing the wrong therapy. Anyhow, that is for another forum. *This* book is to help you prevent your child from suffering at the hands of the mess our healthcare system has become.

The medical system is now disinclined to focus on individual health, and instead is focused on group data and statistical mumbo jumbo such as "quality metrics" and "best practices," none of which have any bearing on what's best for *your* child. If the system continues in this direction, children will be medically managed as if they were all clones.

But your child is special, his asthma is special, and you have every right to want special thought given to your individual child.

If your child receives a "diagnosis" of "asthma," this should immediately raise in your mind the very next question: "What is the *cause* of my child's asthma?"

Asthma is not a specific disease, and it is *not* a diagnosis. It is a reason to search for a diagnosis.

CHAPTER 2

The Physiologic Disturbance of Asthma

Asthma is a physiologic disturbance.

Physiologic means *function*. In the case of asthma, it means *function of the airways*.

Disturbance simply means an *abnormality*.

So "physiologic disturbance" is an *abnormality that causes the airways to not function correctly*. The function of the airways is to let air flow in and out of the lungs. That's an important function!

Asthma is a specific physiologic disturbance—a specific *airway dysfunction*. But the definition of "asthma" that most doctors and medical societies use these days is no longer focused on physiology (function), and this has led to substantial confusion as well as misdirection of research money and intellectual resources. I would ask you instead to join me in a definition of asthma that I prefer. This definition is absolutely central to my philosophy of asthma.

The definition I find most useful for asthma is this: *recurrent episodes of reversible airflow limitation in the chest*.

Let's parse that.

Recurrent: The episodes happen repeatedly.

Reversible: An airflow limitation goes away with time or with medication.

Airflow limitation: Air cannot move through the tubes within the lungs as well as it should.

In the chest: It needs to be in the chest. There are airways *above* the chest that can make noises too, but those noises aren't asthma (although they can be confused with asthma easily).

It is the *airflow limitation* that causes a child to have the symptoms of asthma. Or, if the airflow limitation is above the lungs, can cause symptoms that are *confused* with asthma. It is the *recurrent* and *reversible* components that distinguish *asthma* from lung diseases that cause breathing difficulties, such as pneumonia (which is acute and not *recurrent*) and emphysema / chronic bronchitis (which is *persistent* as opposed to *recurrent*, and the airflow limitation is not reversible).

This definition of asthma that I choose is the definition doctors used fifty years ago. It was the right definition then, and I am convinced it still is now. Later, I will present the *modern* definition that I think has kinda messed up doctors' thinking about asthma. Modern medications for treating children who have asthma are miraculous. Modern *definitions* for asthma are not so good.

Again, my preferred definition of asthma is *recurrent episodes of reversible airflow limitation in the chest.*

For now, let's take a moment for a brief experiment, please.

Open your mouth wide, keep it open, and blow.

Please, go ahead and do it. Give it a big, open-mouthed blow.

When you do that, you huff, but there is no whistle.

Now compare that to when you purse your lips and blow, and intentionally whistle. The narrow hole through your lips causes the whistle.

Wheezing (which you may know well if you have a child with asthma) results from airways that are narrowed enough to make whistling sounds. Usually during *asthma exacerbations* (a term used for acute worsening of asthma) there are lots of airways all making whistling sounds at the same time. This is wheezing. It is the difference between a normal airway (like your wide open mouth) and a narrow airway (like your pursed lips when you whistle).

Wheezing that results from any of the *common* forms of asthma should be *heterophonous,* meaning you can hear multiple different pitches all at the same time. It can sound like the string section of an orchestra tuning up before embarking on playing the theme from Star

Wars. High pitches, low pitches, wiggly pitches, all mixed together.... Those are the common asthma sounds.

You know that when you whistle through your lips, you must have them pursed just the right amount in order for the whistle to happen. You can change the pitch of the whistle by changing the airflow and your lips' positions. But if the lips get too loose *or too tight*, or the flow through them isn't just right, there's no whistle sound made. This same thing is true in the lower airways within the chest. The airflow and diameter in an airway may combine to whistle (wheeze), or they may not. One of the airways may get too narrow to allow a whistle, or the flow may be wrong. The point is that if your child is wheezing, it is only a fraction of the narrowed airways that are making the whistling noises. The rest aren't whistling, but that doesn't mean they are all healthy. Many of the other airways also can be, silently, too narrow.

Wheezing can occasionally come from one single airway, and when it does, it can sound like one single tone, just like the whistle from your lips. This is called homophonous or "same tone" wheezing. Beware of homophonous wheezing in your child! It's often not really asthma but something else entirely. We'll get to that later.

CHAPTER 3

What Causes the Airway Narrowing That Leads to Wheezing?

First, a little anatomy. When you breathe in, air goes in through the nose (or the mouth). From the nose, inhaled air passes in front of the adenoid tissue (you can't see adenoids) then behind the palate and the tonsils and the uvula (the little red man dangling from the palate), down through the hypopharynx (the part of the airway where the air and food passage is shared), and through

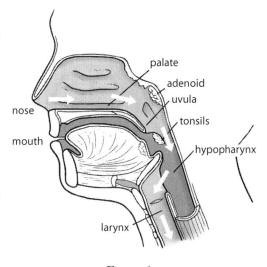

Figure 1

the larynx (voice box) and then into the airways of the chest. It is at the larynx that air is directed into the lungs and food channeled through the esophagus toward the stomach (Figure 1).

This *upper airway* (above the chest) can be narrowed or partially obstructed in several places. The upper airways can therefore make noises of various types, including whistling and wheezing sounds.

17

The noises the upper airways make are very often confused with asthma noises!

The nose can wheeze when congested, especially in infants. Likewise, if the adenoids are swollen for any reason, all sorts of wheezy-type noises can be made. The larynx is a source of lots of wheeze-like noises in infants and children and these are often confused with the noises of asthma, too, because it is often difficult to identify where the noises are coming from.

We will devote a portion of this book to airway noises that frequently get confused with asthma, so that you as a parent are aware of the confusions and can help sort them out (sometimes it is *hard* to sort out).

By the way, upper-airway noises play a big role in older children with asthma who feel like skipping school one day. A school-age child can voluntarily make all sorts of convincing wheezing sounds with very little effort.

Even though some noises that the upper airway makes can *sound* very similar to asthma, the diagnoses and treatments for upper airway noises are entirely different from the diagnoses and treatments for the various causes of asthma. Learning about upper airway noises is particularly important for parents of *younger* children (babies through age 3 years or so), because upper-airway noises are a source of a lot of confusion (confusion with *asthma*) in such little children. More on this topic will follow.

Inside the chest, there are *lots* of airways. The airways that bring air to our lungs are like an upside down tree with multiple branches. And here is something that few people know: the tree-branching pattern is the same in everybody (well, almost everybody). Yes, every child is different in all sorts of ways, but for the most part, their airways all follow nearly identical patterns of branching. *See Figure 2.*

After passing through the larynx into the chest, the air is first inside the *trachea*, which is a single tube. The trachea divides (like an upside down "Y") into the two *mainstem bronchi*, each of which is narrower than the trachea. One bronchus goes to each lung. Off these mainstem bronchi come other airway branches (called *lobar bronchi*) that lead to the three lobes of the lung on the right and the two lobes on the left. These lobar bronchi split into smaller *segmental bronchi* (ten in the right

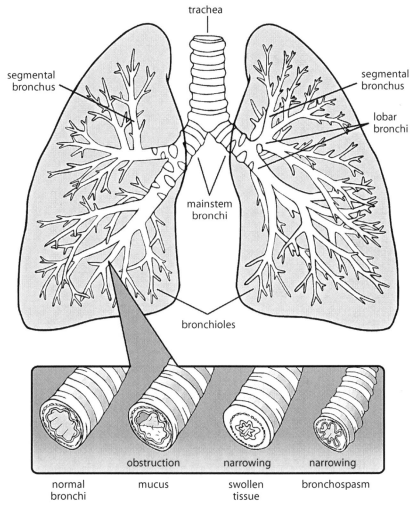

Figure 2

lung and nine in the left lung). These segmental bronchi are all named
and numbered because, again, they have the same pattern in almost
everybody. On their way to the lung tissue itself, these segmental and
subsegmental bronchi keep splitting over and over again into multiple
divisions of smaller airways called *bronchioles*.

Wheezing and other noises can arise in mainstem, lobar, segmental, and subsegmental bronchi and even further down into bronchioles

as the airways keep splitting into smaller and smaller divisions that conduct the air to the microscopic parts of the lungs where the blood and air come together to exchange oxygen and carbon dioxide.

Narrowing and *partial obstruction* of any of these air passages can cause wheezing and other noises. *Complete* narrowing to the point of complete obstruction also occurs. Both the *causes* and the *symptoms* of airway narrowing and obstruction overlap.

Narrowing of the bronchi occurs from three primary causes that often interact.

1. **Bronchospasm**. The bronchial tubes are surrounded by thin layers of muscle. This muscle is supposed to be gently squeezing, just the right amount to help the airways stay circular (which is the shape that air flows through best). If the muscles squeeze down too hard, they can narrow or even close off a bronchial tube. This excessive squeezing can happen from spasm of the muscles: *bronchospasm.* In contrast, if the muscles of the airway are too relaxed (the opposite of bronchospasm), they don't serve their role of keeping the airways circular and the airways can become "floppy" or flattened like a drinking straw that you have chewed on.

> The bronchial-airway muscles are under the control of the same nerves that control the muscles of the body that function automatically (without your thinking about them), like the heart muscle and the muscles in the stomach that churn and digest swallowed food.

2. **Swelling**. The biological tissues that form the airways can become swollen. Inflammation is the most common cause of swelling (but not the only cause). Inflammation is a very important troublemaker in most children with asthma, and so I will have a chapter specifically on inflammation later, and mention it a lot in numerous places in this book. But for now, know that swollen bronchial tissue takes up the space that air is supposed to be moving through, and that means that the air passage is narrowed. It is just like a stuffy nose, but in the lungs: it doesn't matter how hard you blow that stuffy nose, the swollen tissue isn't coming out (only the mucous "boogers" come out).

3. **Small airways.** Some children have smaller airways than other children. Someone has to have smaller-than-average airways, after all. Children with smaller-than-average airways do tend to have more problems with symptoms of narrowed airways. One term to describe this is "congenitally small airways." Congenital just means *at birth*. There is a broad range of normal sizes of airways in children. There is no set cut off for "normal size" and "abnormal size." When airways are narrow (from being very young or very small), even small additional problems (like minor swelling or minor bronchospasm) can cause a whole lot more symptoms from narrowing and obstruction.

4. **Relative narrowing.** Especially if your child happens to be on the lower range of airway size to begin with, whenever he needs to breathe fast (crying, running, feverish, etc.), it may be that the airways then are *relatively* too narrow for the amount of increased air he is trying to move. This *relative narrowing* can lead to asthma symptoms when the need to move air in and out of the lungs is particularly great, even when there is nothing else wrong with his airways.

Obstruction of airways can occur as well, and often occurs along with the narrowing caused by bronchospasm and airway swelling.

1. Most often obstruction is from junk *inside* the airways. Mucus ("boogers") secreted from airway glands is by far the most common culprit, but also bits of sloughed-off cells from the airway wall, bacteria, and pus secreted into the airway can block off the air channels. Sometimes it can be saliva or stomach liquids that have been accidentally breathed down through the larynx. Or it can be mixtures of all of this. Sometimes it is a piece of choked-on food, a toy, or a piece of plastic or something else that just should not be there (a *foreign body*).

2. Sometimes airway obstruction occurs from something compressing an airway from *outside* of it (external to the

airway). The compression can come from lung tissue itself
(particularly lung tissue that is sick and either emptied
of air or overexpanded with air, which causes the airways
nearby to get bent or squeezed). External compression can
be caused by large blood vessels that aren't where they're
supposed to be, and encircle and squeeze an airway. Rarely,
external obstruction of an airway can be caused by areas of
lung infection, swollen lymph nodes near the airways, and
occasionally scary things like tumors.

3. *Partial* obstruction, like narrowing, can lead to noisy airways
(including wheezing). *Complete* obstruction of an airway
however, is *silent*, because there is no airflow through it at all.
This is tricky, isn't it? Sometimes a silent chest is worse than a
wheezy chest. More on that to follow.

A partial obstruction can wheeze like a narrowed airway. A completely obstructed or completely narrowed airway makes no noise.

The noises that emanate from children's airways include sounds other than wheezing. Mucus moving up and down a bronchus can sound like, well, like boogers moving up and down a tube, because that is pretty much what it is. It can be gurgling sounds, juicy sounds, or sounds of nasty wet stuff percolating around.

There are several medical terms that are used to describe the different noises that airways can make, but young and older doctors alike tend to use the informal term "junky sounds" to describe the sounds of wheezing combined with gurgling and popping of mucus moving around within the upper and/or lower airways. And that description is usually adequate, even though not precise. It pretty much means "there are a lot of noises down there and they sound like they are coming from everywhere." So "junky sounds" is a description that is less precise than the term "asthma." Highly experienced physicians still exist who are sticklers for using appropriate terminology for the various breath sounds. But you aren't likely to run into them anymore.

It would be nice if we all had the skill to tell with a stethoscope whether a noise in the chest came from an airway partially obstructed by mucus, or whether it came from an airway narrowed by bronchospasm. But the reality is that the best that even very highly experienced chest physicians can do is to *guess* what we are hearing, and often it is difficult even to know for sure if the noises are coming from the chest as opposed to the upper airway, because the noises can all echo around everywhere.

In the next several chapters, I will go through these various causes of airway narrowing and obstruction. As these causes underlie asthma, they are important to understand. These causes help us to focus in on a diagnosis.

Asthma guidelines used by doctors to manage asthma have classified children as having *intermittent* or *persistent* asthma that is *mild, moderate,* or *severe.* The "official" guidelines have based therapeutic decisions on this categorization. In my opinion, "moderate persistent asthma" is no diagnosis either. It is just a bit of additional description.

I find the terms "mild," "moderate," and "severe" to be of only a little use in childhood asthma. Any of the causes of asthma (any of the underlying diagnoses) can show up at different times as mild, or as moderate, or as severe. In my experience, therapies should be based mostly on the diagnosis, not the severity.

Academic physicians have developed some highly specific criteria for "severe asthma" that other doctors are taught to use. "Severe asthma" has morphed into a diagnostic term (yet it's not!). I don't prefer the complex specific criteria that have been developed.

To me it is pretty simple. Asthma is "severe" if the doctor, parent, or child *thinks* it is severe, and that is the *only* criteria that I use. If it is *severe* in the minds of any of these people in the exam room, then that means we need to put the pedal to the metal to work efficiently toward getting a diagnosis to maximize our chances of making the child better as fast as possible. "Severe asthma" is a reason to work harder and faster to figure out the diagnosis and hone in on the best therapy.

It is important to distinguish *intermittent* from *persistent* asthma.

Intermittent asthma, meaning the asthma goes away completely and comes back, on again and off again, in which a child is *completely* well between episodes, does provide me pretty good reassurance that we are dealing with a common type of asthma that will respond to safe and easy therapies. With intermittent asthma, we have time to sort out the diagnosis (or diagnoses) of the asthma at a conservative and wise pace, without performing unnecessary procedures and spending lots of money. But persistent symptoms that are unrelenting, from which the child never has a day off, means that there is a possibility of a cause that will require more urgent or aggressive treatment (even the possibility of surgery). Therefore obtaining the precise diagnosis (although *always* important in asthma) takes on an urgency in persistent asthma that often requires more frequent office visits, more expenses, and more diagnostic procedures be undertaken.

Persistent asthma may result from any of the common causes of intermittent asthma (and usually does result from the common causes, actually). But sometimes, persistent symptoms result from a foreign body aspirated (inhaled) into the airway that will have to be found and removed, and soon. Or it might rarely come from a tumor in the chest, or it might come from chronic infections associated with significant chronic lung diseases, or several other bad things that we want to know about as soon as we can figure it out.

I want to reiterate that nine times out of ten, persistent asthma is caused by the same diagnoses that cause intermittent asthma, but from which the child just has not had a break. These children will respond well to therapy directed correctly at whatever is causing their asthma (in other words, therapy directed at their diagnosis). But that tenth time, the diagnosis can be very different indeed, and important to find with more haste.

In summary, narrowing and obstruction of airways cause the airflow limitation that leads to many of the symptoms of asthma. Either *persistent* or *severe* asthma are reasons to seek—at a substantially more aggressive pace—the underlying diagnosis of what is causing the asthma.

The next chapters discuss in more detail the various causes of airway narrowing and obstruction.

CHAPTER 4

A Cause of Airflow Narrowing: Bronchospasm

One of the causes of airway narrowing is bronchospasm. The muscles around the airways can squeeze airways closed.

In some ways, bronchospasm is like a muscle cramp in your leg (except it is painless). In any one airway, bronchospasm can happen very fast (closing a small airway in seconds), and if bronchospasm happens in lots of airways in the lungs, it can become symptomatic within a minute or two. The airway muscles can squeeze airways in the mainstem bronchi as well as airways further out in the periphery of the lung.

Bronchospasm can happen when the airways get tickled. So let's talk about ticklishness for a moment. I'll start with an analogy: tickling feet.

Ticklishness of the bottom of a foot depends on a few things:

1. The nature of the object touching the foot. A feather will tickle; the sole of a shoe does not tickle.
2. The sensitivity of the nerves of the foot. Some people are ticklish, and some people just aren't. How many nerves there are, and the types of nerves, are determinants of ticklishness.
3. How long the tickling has gone on. The ticklishness can go away if the bottom of the foot is touched for long enough.

I am not trying to frighten you, but it is true that the speed at which bronchospasm can narrow airways is one of the frightening things about asthma. The reality is that very, very few children die from asthma, and if you understand asthma, your child is very, very unlikely to be one of those.

25

4. The emotional state of the tickled person. Sometimes a person is ticklable, and sometimes they just aren't.

Of course, the consequences of ticklishness in the airways is more troublesome than a tickled foot. That is why asthma brings people to doctors, but foot ticklishness does not. Even so, the comparison to foot ticklishness is helpful. When the foot is tickled, the muscles contract to protect the foot from the tickling object. When something tickles the airway, the muscles of the airway contract to protect the lungs from the tickling object. In people who have asthma, those airway muscles sometimes respond excessively.

Let's say the tickling object in the airway is a piece of feather that has escaped from a pillow. A feather in the airway can lead to infections and trouble, so it is something we do not want there. As the feather touches an airway wall, a nerve senses it and sends signals to the airway muscles to squeeze down and narrow that airway, perhaps to help prevent more feathers from being sucked into it. This is good behavior of the airway muscles. Signals also go to your central nervous system that tell you to cough to try to expel the feather. Such coughing and bronchospasm are protective for you.

But the airways can get too ticklish. Too many sensory nerves can be there, and those nerves may make a mistake and misinterpret something otherwise pretty harmless, like dry air, as if it were a feather. Or they may interpret a harmless bit of small booger passing by as if the booger were something more dangerous (like a tiny piece of aspirated Lego or a peanut). And if this misinterpretation happens, the muscles of the airway will respond by squeezing, and your child may cough and wheeze, even though the dry air or small booger are no danger to the airway, and there is really no foreign object like a feather, Lego, or peanut to expel. This hypersensitivity of the nerves to airway stimulation can lead to inappropriate bronchospasm and airway narrowing and "asthma" in many people. This hypersensitivity is called *bronchial hyperreactivity* and it is a very common component of children's asthma, so common in fact that the most careful respiratory specialist doctors won't "diagnose" asthma without bronchial hyperreactivity being present. In reality, few doctors formally test for bronchial hyperreactivity in patients with asthma. It is such a common component of most asthma that it is just assumed to be present, based on a patient's history. However, testing for bronchial hyperreactivity more regularly would help us all understand what sorts of lung diseases children have.

I used the word "diagnose" just then in that previous paragraph. But please don't forget, asthma is not really a diagnosis.

It may not be the sensory nerves that are messing up to cause bronchospasm. It may be the muscles that are overly twitchy. They may sense a small and normal nerve signal and instead of squeezing slightly to adjust the airway size slightly, they may spasm down like an angry dog barking at the postman—in other words, an unnecessary overreaction.

Either the nerves being too sensitive or the muscles being too twitchy (or both together) leads to bronchial hyperreactivity. Bronchial hyperreactivity means that the airways overreact to stimulation, and go into bronchospasm. They are overly ticklish and overly twitchy airways.

Dry air is indeed one of the triggers that causes hyperreactive bronchi to spasm. It is one of the most important triggers of lower-airway narrowing (asthma) in *exercise-induced asthma*. After a few minutes of running, a child (whether asthmatic or not) will change from breathing through her nose to breathing through her mouth so she can move more air and get more oxygen to her muscles. The nose cannot move as much air as the mouth can, but the nose is *much* better than the mouth at humidifying inhaled air. So when mouth breathing starts during exercise, poorly humidified dry air from the mouth gets down into the chest airways, and if those airways are twitchy and ticklish, the nerves sense the dry air, mistake it for a feather, and bronchospasm can result. *That is* exercise-induced asthma. By the way, the air breathed through the mouth is also not warmed as well as air breathed through the nose, and some children's airways are likely twitchy in response to cold air, as well as dry air. Often dry and cold air go hand in hand. More will follow about exercise-induced asthma later in this book.

Next is a slightly more complicated cause of bronchospasm. Inhalation of chlorine gas from just above the water in a pool, or from household bleach, can trigger the airway nerves to prompt bronchospasm. This happens because the chlorine gas dissolves into the thin layer of watery fluid that lines and lubricates all the airways, and it acidifies this *airway lining fluid*. The airway doesn't like acid in it any more than your eye appreciates it if acidic lemon juice is squirted into it, and the airway reacts with anger, including, among other things, bronchospasm. Some children are more sensitive to acid inhalation than others, and respond with more bronchospasm and cough. Unlike the response to dry air, though, acid can cause lots of injuries to the airway, so the airway has developed lots of responses to acid beyond just bronchospasm, such as inflammation and mucus secretion. We'll get to those later.

All children are different, and some can tolerate small amounts of acid inhalation without injury at all, and without bronchospasm or cough. Other children will suffer some degree of airway injury and/or airway bronchospasm or cough with even tiny amounts of acid in the airway. And here's another trick to know: children change. Your child might tolerate a bit of chlorine exposure at one point without any problem, but then later not tolerate it at all and cough and wheeze a lot. Immunologic and nerve changes that occur in the lung from other causes, including viral infections, may change the way a child responds to stuff that gets in the lungs, and these changes may occur over years, or even week to week. Asthma is often a variable and changing physiologic disturbance that shows up with a variable degree of symptoms—sometimes bad, sometimes barely a bother at all.

By the way, breathing in some acidic stomach contents ("aspiration"), even in teeny tiny amounts, can cause the airways to respond with bronchospasm, cough, mucus secretion, and inflammation. Stomach acid getting into the airways is a problem for some children with asthma, sometimes, but not all children, and not always. More on this issue in subsequent chapters.

Cold, dry air as a cause of bronchospasm is a relatively simple thing to understand. And obviously the airway is going to respond to acid getting inhaled into it. Other ways that bronchospasm can occur are a bit more complex—with interacting cellular, physical and chemical pathways. Here is one example, and an example that will introduce you to a key concept—*inflammation.*

Let's say that your child is allergic to dust mites, or to pollen, or to pet dander. And a bit of that allergen gets inhaled into his chest. If that

Dander is mostly bits of skin flakes from your pet.

tiny microscopic bit of allergen lands on an airway wall near certain types of immunologic cells, those cells can spit out chemical signals to the other cells in the airway. *Bronchospasm* is *one* of the many responses of the airway to the signals released from the cells. So inhalation of allergens to which your child is allergic can cause bronchospasm.

When allergens cause bronchospasm, you can count on them causing lots of inflammation as well. And the more inflammation there is, the more likely that an inhaled allergen will come in contact with one of those immune cells that tells the airways to bronchospasm. So allergic inflammation leads to more bronchial hyperreactivity. We will talk plenty about inflammation in the next chapter (and beyond). Inflammation is *very* important in *most* (but *not* all) children with asthma.

Bronchospasm in children can be triggered by inhaled allergens or irritants (including cigarette smoke and wood smoke), and also by emotional stress, hormonal fluctuations, stomach acid reflux into the esophagus, aspiration of saliva or stomach fluid, viral infections and bacterial infections.

Bronchospasm may have developed to help protect our lungs from bad exposures. But in people who have asthma, very often that protection is worse than the exposure. The protective mechanism becomes the danger to us. In this way it is like a child being tickled (not dangerous) who kicks around wildly and smashes his leg into a lamp (injurious).

When it comes to bronchospasm, where possible (and it is not always possible) it is helpful to find out what seems to trigger it in *your* child, and deal with those exposures to the extent you can.

No paranoia is needed here. I am not recommending preventing your child from exercising, from breathing through his mouth, from doing cleaning chores that involve bleach, from swimming in a pool or sitting around a campfire. Rather, I am suggesting that you watch to see what *might* cause problems, and help your child through them with gentle combinations of avoidance, medications, and other tools.

And this raises another key point. Successful management of asthma means that asthma barely interferes with your child's life beyond a few minutes a day. Successful management of asthma means that your child's choices in life are not limited by asthma except in a few small and mostly innocuous ways. Even scuba diving is possible for well-managed asthmatics to undertake (but only under careful guidance of an experienced scuba doctor!). Successful management of asthma is not focused on fear and avoidance, but on preparation for and enjoyment of all that life can offer. It's a philosophical concept. Don't focus on fear. Focus on opportunity!

CHAPTER 5

Inflammation as a Cause of Airway Narrowing

Another cause of airway narrowing is *inflammation*. I have mentioned inflammation several times, because it is a very important component to address in most children with asthma.

Inflammatory cells take up space within the airway. Inflammation expands the bulk of tissue of the airway wall (which encroaches upon the air channels in airways, *narrowing* the airway and limiting airflow). Inflammatory cells release compounds that cause more damage to the airway tissues and that increase the twitchiness/ticklishness of airways (increasing bronchospasm). Inflammation can lead to all manners of airway dysfunction.

In most (but not all) patients, most of the time (but not all of the time), inflammation ends up being the worst troublemaker in children with asthma.

In fact, inflammation is so commonly important that the medical community collectively (and against my wishes, what d'ya know!) decided to incorporate "inflammation" into the modern definition of asthma. (Remember, I don't like the modern definition, and this incorporation of *inflammation* into the definition is the main reason why I don't.)

The modern definition of asthma goes something like this: "a chronic inflammatory airway disease that leads to recurrent episodes of reversible airway narrowing and bronchial hyperreactivity." There is a lot of overlap of this with my preferred definition, but the problem with the modern definition is that it limits "asthma" as a term only to

When you see the four letters "-itis" at the end of an anatomic term of some kind, it means *inflammation*. "Bronchitis" thus means *inflammation of the bronchi*; laryngitis means *inflammation of the larynx*. It is important to note that "-itis" does not tell you what caused the inflammation. It might be a bacterial infection resulting in inflammation, or it might not. It might be a viral infection, or it might not. It might be allergic inflammation, or it might not. All "-itis" means is that there is *inflammation of some kind*. And, if therapy is needed, the therapy will depend on the cause and type of the inflammation. Any word with "-itis" at the end of it is not a diagnosis any more than *asthma* is, but rather a reason to look for a diagnosis.

be used if there is airway inflammation present. In fact, inflammation is a central component, a sine qua non, of this *modern* diagnosis of "asthma" (remember, I think "asthma" is not a diagnosis!).

Here is one problem with the modern definition: very rarely is airway inflammation actually ever measured in patients with asthma; so the doctors don't know if it is there, or, if it *is* present, how much inflammation there is. So how can inflammation be included in the definition of "asthma" that doctors are told to use, when in any individual patient with asthma they don't actually know if inflammation is present?

And here is another trick. Inflammation is a *very* nebulous and *very* complex term that incorporates hundreds of chemicals, hundreds of cell types, thousands of proteins, and all sorts of other biological components as well as the myriad of interactions amongst them all. Inflammation as a whole is a broad concept, and therefore quantifying inflammation is fraught with misleading measurements.

There are all sorts of very different types of inflammation. Your child's airways might be highly inflamed based on *one* measure of "inflammation" while another measurement of some other chemical or cell shows no inflammation at all! Inflammation incited by viral infections is different from inflammation that arises in response to bacterial infections. Inflammation from allergies is different from the inflammation that follows injuries. Certain types of inflammation are closely associated with asthma and can be considered causative of asthma symptoms, and other types of inflammation are not at all associated with asthma symptoms.

I do not believe the term "inflammation" belongs in the definition of asthma for several reasons: 1) because doctors rarely measure any of the types of inflammation in patients with asthma; 2) because inflammation has so many *different* types; 3) because inflammation is not always present in patients who wheeze and cough and who get "diagnosed" with asthma.

So I will stick to my physiologic, non-immunologic definition of asthma, which if you recall is *recurrent episodes of reversible airflow limitation in the chest.*

And now I reiterate that various types of inflammation are critically important in *most* children who have asthma. So, just because inflammation isn't in my definition of asthma, doesn't mean I don't think inflammation is very important to consider and to deal with.

I mentioned that inflammation is hard to define. There is an old Latin definition that is the best I know of. Inflammation is a combination of:

- *Rubor* (redness): Usually comes from increased blood flow.
- *Tumor* (swelling): Not to be confused with the modern English term "tumor" that means a mass or growth. *Tumor (swelling)* can arise from increased blood flow, fluid leakage into tissue, or accumulation of immunologic cells within the tissue.
- *Calor* (heat): Usually from increased blood flow or increased tissue metabolism.
- *Dolor* (pain): From nerves being stimulated by chemicals released from injured cells.

In the inflamed airways, these four Latin terms all occur (although the airway doesn't translate *dolor* as pain, but rather as ticklishness or an itch, or a desire to cough).

The body responds to all sorts of injuries and infections with various types of inflammation that usually help destroy invading infections, or help the body to heal; but sometimes the inflammation is mistaken, excessive, misdirected, or outright stupid, and then the inflammation

By the way, what is an itch? This is cool. The formal medical definition for "itch" is "a sensation that prompts a desire to scratch." Brilliant, huh? Actually it makes sense. In the airway, an "itch" prompts the desire to *cough*. Coughing scratches the itch in the airways. Remember that old adage: *"The more you itch, the more you scratch. The more you scratch the more you itch."* That applies in the lungs as well. A quick way to make the lungs get all itchy (and inflamed) is to start coughing unnecessarily. The more you cough, the more you itch.

itself *causes* injuries to us instead of healing injuries.

In most but not all children with asthma, inflammation gets stupid and injures the child's airway, which leads to symptoms of asthma.

This is worth repeating with different words. *In most children with asthma, excessive, misdirected, or unnecessary inflammation causes (or substantially contributes to) the physiologic disturbance and symptoms of asthma.*

How can we know if inflammation is present in *your* child's airway? Well, it really *is* hard to know. It is hard to measure airway inflammation.

Is your child's airway red (*rubor*)? Who knows? We can place a tube with a camera deep down into the lungs to look and see, but that's no fun for anybody. I have enormous experience looking into children's bronchi and I can assure you that determining if an airway is mildly red is pretty much guesswork. I don't recommend it.

Is your child's airway swollen (*tumor*— remember this means the *Latin* "tumor," not the English "tumor")? Well, we can guess about it a bit. We at least can usually tell if there is *narrowing* (which can come from inflammation or from bronchospasm or other reasons) by listening for wheezing. Or we can seek the presence of narrowing and obstruction by doing special measurements of airflow called *spirometry*. And we can do more extensive testing called *plethysmography* that can distinguish narrowing from obstruction. And with these tests, along with use of medications that relax airway muscles, we can make good guesses as to whether airway narrowing is from the swelling or just from bronchospasm. But we still wouldn't know that the swelling is from inflammation.

Is your child's airway hot (*calor*)? I won't get into it in detail, but we haven't really figured out how to measure airway temperature in a way that is clinically helpful. People are working on it. For now, *calor* doesn't help in our assessment of airway inflammation.

Is your child's airway itchy (*dolor*)? This is the easiest thing to tell. When children itch, they scratch. When airways itch, children cough. So when your child coughs it means her airway nerves are itching, and one of the causes of airway itching is inflammation. But cough can happen without inflammation at all. For example, when a child coughs from inhalation of chlorine or aspiration of stomach acid, or a booger that gets too big in the airway, then the cough comes from a protective reflex nerve response, not from inflammation.

Overall, even the most comprehensive definition of inflammation we have—*rubor, tumor, calor, dolor*—is only minimally useful to your doctor in terms of determining whether there is inflammation present.

What *can* your doctor do to test for inflammation in airways?

There are many scientists doing research to figure this out, because, gee, if we could actually measure airway inflammation and parse out the different types of inflammation easily, then we could use such measurements to help diagnose the causes of asthma and learn how to treat inflammation better in each individual child. Right now there are only a couple of ways to measure inflammation in clinical settings outside of research hospitals.

Exhaled nitric oxide. Nitric oxide is a gas that is formed in the airways. It is but one of the myriad components of inflammation, but it does roughly correlate with *allergic* types of inflammation in the lungs (but not other types of inflammation). It is pretty easy to measure now (after a lot of research, engineering, and money went into it). It is a simple measure performed on an exhaled breath! Exhaled nitric oxide levels provide some help in diagnosing causes of asthma symptoms, and can provide some help in managing asthma too. A minority of lung specialists will have the capability of measuring exhaled nitric oxide in your child, and exceedingly few pediatricians or family-practice doctors will be able to do it. But it *can* be done. It is not the end all and be all of diagnostic tests, however, so if your doctor doesn't offer it, that's okay. It is also really tough to get the measurement accomplished in children under 6 years old.

Sputum cell counts. Sputum is the goobers that get coughed up from the lower airways (below the vocal cords/larynx). Sputum gets mixed with boogers from the nose and saliva from the mouth and secretions from the esophagus, so it is a messy sample that arises from everywhere in the whole airway, not just the lungs. But if a big loogey of sputum gets coughed up by your child in a clinic, it is often worthwhile to have technicians or doctors look at it under the microscope in a lab to identify the inflammatory/immunologic cells that are in it. This microscopic evaluation can determine if there is cellular inflammation present and if so, what type of inflammation it might be (such as whether it is an allergic inflammation, or an inflammation that is fighting a viral infection or bacterial infection).

It is a challenge to get sputum from children. Particularly when asthma is mild or stable, children often don't cough up sputum. Sputum in older children can be "induced" or "encouraged" in a doctor's office for the purpose of getting a sample. Unfortunately, this technique is not commonly available even in specialist offices. If you happen to find a doctor that will induce and analyze sputum cell counts to assess inflammation, that's a special doctor. It is one of the most useful tests to diagnose what is causing a patient's asthma, and therefore one of the most helpful tests for managing difficult-to-control asthma.

Without performing any tests for inflammation at all (the overwhelmingly usual reality), we are left with guessing about what type of lung inflammation might be present. And it turns out that, absent laboratory tests, the best way we have to guess about what type of inflammation might be present is to *diagnose the cause of the asthma*.

Thus, in the typical doctor's office where no testing is done for airway inflammation, doctors usually end up guessing whether inflammation is present and what type of inflammation it might be. We can get help with our guessing from some of the best medical minds of the past hundred years and today, from the huge amounts of research into asthma they have undertaken, and their extensive clinical experience.

I would like to present a very small sample of what we have learned (so far) about inflammation because it will help in understanding how medications work for different types of asthma.

Allergic inflammation often involves (among many others) a cell type called *eosinophils*. Eosinophils seem to have developed to fight against parasitic infections (like intestinal worms), which to this day are extremely common infestations of children in less-developed countries. Eosinophils were designed to bury inside the worms and release enzymes and oxidants inside them to kill the worm. If eosinophils accumulate where there are no worms, they can try to burrow their way into other things, like the thin lining of our airway walls, where they release their enzymes and oxidants causing injury and airway dysfunction and more inflammation. Eosinophils disappear rapidly and cleanly when patients are treated with steroid medications.

Allergic inflammation also often includes *mast cells*. Mast cells accumulate within the tissue that lines the mucous membranes, in the eye, the airway, and the digestive system, as well as in the skin. Mast cells also have a role in fighting parasites, but are now more well-known for the very rapid allergic response that happens when a mast cell comes in contact with something to which your child has developed an allergic sensitivity. Mast cells release compounds (including histamine) that cause itchy eyes, sneezing, coughing, and bronchospasm (and diarrhea in the gut, and hives in the skin). It is allergically sensitized mast cells that allergists are seeking when they perform allergy skin tests on a child. Mast cells play a very big role in acute allergic reactions, including *anaphylactic shock.*

There are many other cell types centrally involved in allergic inflammation as well. *Allergic inflammation* often plays a primary role in asthma, and when it does, the diagnosis of *allergic inflammatory asthma* is appropriate. I will use that diagnostic term a lot.

Anti-infective inflammation. There are many immunologic cells involved in fighting off infections. A cell type called the *neutrophil* is an evolutionarily ancient immune cell whose job includes fighting bacteria, so neutrophils tend to come into an airway that the neutrophils assume (rightly or wrongly) has a bacterial infection. They also accumulate in certain stages of viral respiratory infections of the airway. They migrate toward areas that are acidic, too. Neutrophils make up much of pus. They release an enzyme—designed to help make oxidants to fight infections—that is green in color, and this is the main reason why pus is green. Yuk. Now, neutrophils are not smart cells! Neutrophils can injure your own tissue with the same chemicals and enzymes that they use to try to kill off infectious organisms. Unlike the eosinophils of allergic inflammation, neutrophils do *not* go away when a patient is treated with steroid medications. Indeed, steroids actually can encourage neutrophils to stick around longer and cause more problems.

There are other types of inflammation as well, but this information so far is enough to make an important point. Please remember that inhaled steroid medication—a fantastically wonderful medication that helps so many children with asthma—will reduce allergic inflammation, but won't reduce, and may even worsen, inflammation from infections.

CHAPTER 6

Obstruction of Airways: Glandular Secretions (Mucus 'n' Boogers), Pus, Inhaled Dust, and Other Goo

Obstruction of an airway (and remember there are lots of airways) can be partial or complete. In terms of how air can pass through, the effect of partial obstruction is very similar to the effect of narrowing. In turn, bronchospasm and inflammation can sometimes narrow an airway all the way to closure (complete obstruction). Narrowing and obstruction occur together in patients who have asthma symptoms.

Obstruction of an airway can be caused by accumulation of glandular secretions. The airways in the chest have glands that secrete mucus very much like the nose does. When your nose gets a cold, or an allergy, the nasal tissue (1) gets inflamed (swollen) and it also (2) secretes more glandular mucus. The same thing happens in the airways of the chest.

You can blow your nose to temporarily clear out nasal mucus ("boogers" in the parlance of children and pediatricians), but the boogers re-accumulate pretty fast. You *cannot* blow out the swollen nasal tissue, no matter how hard you try (and blowing a nose hard actually just makes the nasal tissue *more* swollen). In the lung you can cough up the mucus, but it can be a lot harder to accomplish than clearing a nose. The mucus in the lungs is deeper, for one thing. Also, for clearing the nose, you can squeeze one nostril closed and have your child blow through the other nostril to get boogers out. But you can't do the same with a lung!

Healthy airways in the chest are lined with microscopic hairs (called *cilia*) that move in a coordinated fashion to propel normal airway fluid as well as trapped inhaled particles and secreted mucus up higher and higher in the airway, up through the segmental bronchi, up through the lobar bronchi, up through the mainstem bronchi, up through the trachea, and through and out of the larynx. (At which point your child will unconsciously swallow the yucky stuff down into the stomach—which is fine, by the way. It won't hurt the little guy, and there isn't much you can do to teach a child how to hock it out into a tissue, so I recommend not stressing over it. Let him swallow his snot.)

Cilia do their job pretty slowly, but when the airway is sick, the cilia may not do their job at all. When cilia aren't doing their job, mucus gets stuck down there in the airways of the chest. Cilia have trouble doing their job when there are viruses or bacteria in the airway, when allergic inflammation (including eosinophils and mast cells) have released toxins that injure the cilia cells, when the airway is acidic, or when exposed to excessive smoke, among other causes.

Also, when there are viruses, bacteria, allergic exposures, acid exposures, or smoke inhalation, the glands of the airway respond by secreting more mucus. The mucus builds up and it soon triggers in airway nerves some *dolor* (ticklishness), which causes us to reflexively cough to try to force the mucus out. Coughing can generate *really* high pressures in the lungs to try to blow out the accumulated gunk.

With bacterial and viral infections, pus cells hang out with the glandular secretions too, alongside bits of injured airway-lining cells (called *epithelial cells*) that the infection, inflammation, toxin, or acid insult has sickened. Also in the mucus are microscopic particles of inhaled stuff that the cilia are supposed to be clearing out.

I would bet you have sat near a window through which a bright beam of sunlight has shone, and stared at all the sparkling bits that float in the air and catch and reflect the sunlight. It is beautiful. It's a sunbeam! Your child probably has great fun wiggling his hand through, or blowing through, the sunbeam to stir up the sparkles and make them dance.

Those sparkles are dust, and they are floating in the air whether or not there is a sunbeam to reveal them.

When your child breathes through her nose, the nose filters out most of the visible reflective particles, so that they don't get into the lungs. But where there are reflective particles (big enough to see in a sunbeam), you can be sure there are invisible microscopic particles as well, and lots of them. A nose is not as good at filtering out *microscopic* particles, so when they are breathed in, some go straight on through into the lung. The lung secretions capture them and the cilia clear them out. At least that is the way it works when all is healthy.

Do not live in paranoid fear of inhaling particles from the air. Our healthy body is designed to deal with most of them. But these particles *are* relevant in certain settings, particularly if your child is allergic to some of the stuff in the dust. We will have a whole chapter on the allergies to microscopic bits of stuff that children (and you) inhale.

The nutshell is that in the airways of the chest, there are secretions from glands, pus, bits of airway-lining cells, and inhaled dust that all can accumulate. If this stuff gets into the airway faster than the cilia can clear it, coughing takes over to help get rid of it. If coughing isn't able to clear it, the accumulating goo begins to obstruct whichever of the airways it is in. And that limits airflow and contributes to asthma (*recurrent, reversible airflow limitation in the chest*).

And speaking of nutshells, an airway can get obstructed by inhaling a nutshell into it, or a whole nut, or gum, or a gum wrapper, or a toy, or a grape, or any of lots of other things. In small children, you might have no clue that they choked on something and breathed it into their airway. If it is big, an inhaled foreign body can get stuck at the vocal cords or just below them and cause extreme and immediate danger requiring clearance (such as using back blows, abdominal thrusts, or the Heimlich maneuver). However, if small enough, the foreign object will fall down into just one of several smaller airways, and immediate life-threatening problems might be avoided, but the foreign object *will* cause trouble pretty soon. A foreign object in an airway is one of the problems that can cause a homophonous wheeze (single-tone wheeze), as opposed to the typical asthmatic multiple-tone wheeze. Or it can completely occlude (fully obstruct) an airway and *silently* lead to real problems in the lung tissue behind it, including pneumonias.

A foreign object in the airway is something that we always have to think about in children who have funny or different wheezing, or multiple pneumonias, or who don't follow a usual pattern. And always in a child who has a new lung disease and a history of choking on something. It is the experienced physician who is best in a position to help you figure this out. This is one reason why it is indeed so important to work with a physician as the diagnosis for your child's asthma is sorted out. Guessing if there is a foreign body in a lung requires experience and often x-rays or placing a camera in the chest airways (*bronchoscopy*) for an examination. As the old warning goes: "Don't do this at home."

If asthma is not getting better after diagnosis is established and appropriate interventions undertaken, somewhere on the list of potentially confounding issues should be the question: "Might my child have choked on something that's still down there?"

CHAPTER 7

Obstruction of an Airway from Something Outside the Airway That Compresses or Kinks It

The airways in the chest are like upside down branches of trees, and the leaves on those tree branches would be the lung tissue where air and blood come together to exchange oxygen for carbon dioxide. In the lung, the leaves aren't flat and instead are more like little bags of air—actually tiny little balloons or sacs.

This next bit is scary sounding, but don't let it scare you. If an airway is completely obstructed for any reason, the air in those tiny balloons or sacs of lung gets absorbed by the passing bloodstream. Because no fresh new air can get to them during breathing, the sacs deflate. All the little air sacs beyond an obstructed airway slowly become empty. When this happens, the whole part of the lung beyond the obstructed airway empties. The medical term for this area of noninflated lung tissue is *atelectasis*. The common lay term that sounds more scary is *lung collapse*.

The volume of a collapsed part of the lung can shrink to 20% of its normal air-filled volume. And as it shrinks, it tugs on the airway that feeds it, contorting the airway or twisting it. Even if the obstruction in the airway comes free, it can take a while for the airway to reopen, and to refill those air sacs back up.

More rarely, a pneumonia or abscess can compress adjacent airways and squeeze them closed, partially or completely. Much rarer still, a tumor in the lung or lymph nodes can do this also. An enlarged lymph node from infection or other major inflammation can squeeze adjacent airways as well.

I frequently say that everybody is different. Everybody *is* different in various ways, and that is why one-size-fits-all notions in health care decisions, health insurance, and health policy do every individual child a disservice sooner or later. I mentioned earlier that the airways follow a branching pattern that is very similar in *almost* everyone, but not everyone. The same is true of the large blood vessels that carry blood flow out of the heart to the head and body and lungs. Sometimes (fortunately rarely) a large blood vessel forms incorrectly during fetal development and loops around and compresses the trachea, or any of the larger bronchi. This causes an external compression that narrows or obstructs an airway and leads to wheezing and other symptoms. This sort of wheezing is often monophonous (single tone), but not always.

An abnormally located large blood vessel that squeezes an airway is one of several very different causes of an airway disorder called *malacia*. Malacia is commonly confused with asthma-type symptoms. It is convenient to talk about it next.

CHAPTER 8

Malacia

What on earth is *malacia*? It is most probably an entirely unfamiliar term to you. Yet all it is is a highfalutin' medical term for *floppy*. Malacia, malacia, malacia. Please say it a few times. Now, say "floppy airway, floppy airway, floppy airway." Malacia is a "floppy airway." Don't let an unknown word cause your attention to fade. Malacia equals floppy.

Please play with your ear for a moment: bend it around, wiggle it. There is cartilage in your ear that helps your ear maintain its shape. This sort of cartilage is firm, but flexible. It holds its shape mostly, but bends if you want to bend it.

The bigger airways (trachea and bronchi) are held open in part by cartilage that is similar to the cartilage that keeps the shape of your ear. Usually the airway cartilage does a fine job keeping the airways round and open for best airflow.

Floppy airways are airways in which the muscle and the firmer cartilage that are supposed to keep the airway's round shape aren't doing their jobs. The cartilage may be thin, wimpy, or incompletely formed. Or it may have been compressed by a blood vessel that formed in slightly the wrong place.

The big airways (trachea and mainstem bronchi) have cartilage that encircles most of the airway. The back sides of the airways are softer membranes with less cartilage. Particularly if the airway cartilage is weak, coughing—or even just hard breathing through a congested nose—can cause the membrane in the back of the airway to bow forward and momentarily obstruct the airway. The noises that can be made when this happens are remarkable (*very* "junky" noises), and these noises can and do get confused with "asthma."

45

Malacia usually is present at birth and noticed soon thereafter, and, as long as there is not something else wrong (such as a blood vessel in the wrong place), malacia gradually goes away as the cartilage normally strengthens over time.

There are several anatomic locations in which malacia can occur.

Laryngomalacia is floppiness of the cartilage in the voice box. It is the most common type of malacia. It can be mild and an occasional nuisance, or it can be very severe and disrupt breathing to the point that a baby cannot eat easily and cannot gain weight. It shows up with really noisy breathing and a baby that works hard to breathe intermittently.

Here's a trick: laryngomalacia shows up with *recurrent episodes of reversible airflow obstruction*, which means it is a lot like asthma (which only has the addition of "*in the chest*" in its definition). But laryngomalacia is actually *above* the chest. Identifying the precise location of narrowing or obstruction is hard for either you or your doctor to do, so laryngomalacia can get confused with various types of asthma and other breathing problems. *You* are now aware of laryngomalacia, and your awareness will help you and your doctor consider the possibility. Most pediatricians and family practitioners are also aware of laryngomalacia.

Laryngomalacia can cause wheezing noises that get confused with various types of asthma, but the sounds of laryngomalacia are usually coarser and rougher and gooier than the wheezing that occurs from asthma.

Laryngomalacia is usually more symptomatic when a baby is lying on his back and/or is busy or excited or upset. Placing a baby that has laryngomalacia on his belly helps to open up his airway and helps him breathe easier. This little trick helps us to *diagnose* laryngomalacia. And keeping a baby on his belly *while awake* can be a cautious part of the *therapy* for laryngomalacia.

Good news about laryngomalacia: it usually goes away on its own by 6 to 12 months of age. But that depends on normal growth of the baby and that the malacia not be too severe. Infants with severe laryngomalacia may need high tech assistance for a time to help them breathe until their laryngomalacia gets better.

Medications used for asthma do no good for laryngomalacia.

Tracheomalacia is floppiness of the airway cartilage in the trachea—the big tube in the center of the chest below the larynx. The back of the trachea is always a bit floppy, but in some children the back of the trachea is overly floppy or the front or sides of the airway are floppy also. Tracheomalacia causes lots of breathing noises too. It occurs along with laryngomalacia in some children, shows up with noisy breathing and coughing when an infant gets upset or really excited, or when exerting herself (such as running around, in the older infant/toddler). Tracheomalacia also usually gets better on its own over time (by 18 months).

Bronchomalacia is floppiness of the first couple of divisions of the lower airways beyond the trachea, and can very much sound like the wheezing that can be confused with so many various causes of asthma. Indeed, bronchomalacia is a cause of recurrent episodes of airflow limitation, but they aren't rapidly *reversible*. Bronchomalacia usually is associated with some degree of laryngomalacia and tracheomalacia. It takes a couple of years for it to get better, but those years can be tough. Anti-inflammatory medications and bronchial-muscle-relaxing medications (such as most of the medications used today for asthma) *do not work for bronchomalacia*, and actually may make the problem worse. It takes a wise parent and a wise doctor to come together to think about the possibility of bronchomalacia as the cause of a baby's noisy breathing. Now you know that

Note that there are *strong* recommendations by medical experts that young babies should *sleep* on their *backs*, and *not* their bellies. This advice is to decrease the risk of Sudden Infant Death Syndrome (SIDS, or "crib death") and indeed it is very effective at lowering the risk of SIDS deaths. The campaign to get babies to sleep on their backs has wonderfully decreased the number of SIDS deaths. However, the recommendations to have a baby sleep on her back are, once again, guidelines written for the average baby, and not specifically for the babies with laryngomalacia. If your baby has laryngomalacia, the data about SIDS and sleeping position in general do not *directly* apply, and you should sit down with your doctor to find out what makes the most sense as far as sleeping position for your baby.

bronchomalacia exists, and this knowledge may be enough to help your child. A confident diagnosis of bronchomalacia can best be made by a pediatric pulmonologist.

Malacia is mostly a problem in infants. Again, it is just like the ear. A newborn baby's ear is *really* floppy, and sometimes his airways can be too. The ear gets firmer as a child grows older, and so do the airways.

Until the cartilage strengthens (over the first year or two of life), if your baby has malacia at any level (larynx, trachea, or bronchi), count on really noisy breathing whenever any of the following occurs:

1. Your baby is sad or mad. Crying makes malacia very apparent.
2. Your baby has some lung disease—pneumonia, viral bronchiolitis, or other cause of lung or airway inflammation—and is working hard to breathe. Malacia makes infants have to work even harder.
3. Your baby has a fever and is breathing fast as a result.
4. Your baby has a congested (stuffy) nose. Airway malacia is more symptomatic when airflow through the nose is narrowed from a cold, or from crying, or other causes of nasal obstruction.
5. Your baby is really happy and excited and busy.

In all of these settings, malacia is more likely to be apparent and troublesome. Note that malacia can be noisy even when your child is otherwise completely well and as happy as a camper, if he is excited and breathing more air as a result of that excitement. A "very happy wheezer" makes me think that a child might have malacia.

As I mentioned, medications don't do much to help malacia. In fact, excessive use of bronchodilator medications (a type of medication discussed in chapter 27) can even make malacia worse. Some gentle airway muscle tension helps provide support in the wimpy malacic airway, and bronchodilator medications may relax the airway muscle too much.

Again, the malacic airway gradually improves on its own as cartilage thickens over months to a year or two or three, and the symptoms will subside. This is very fortunate, as we have no medical interventions that work to make it better. As I mentioned before, sometimes we need to provide high tech medical devices to help a baby breathe until she outgrows her condition. Such therapy would be handled by a pediatric pulmonologist and/or a pediatric otolaryngologist (ear/nose/throat doctor, also known as an ENT physician).

There are exceptions to the spontaneous improvement of malacia as a child gets older. There is another cause of asthma-like symptoms that occurs from an anatomic mistake that sometimes occurs during fetal development. It is rare and usually identified in the first year of life. In some children, the esophagus and the trachea (or a bronchus) are connected by a fistula (a tissue tube that shouldn't be there) and food from the esophagus can get into the airway through this tube. This is a big problem and needs diagnosis and surgical removal of that improper connection. But after the surgery, the airway involved is often left overly floppy (malacic) and it can take many years of patience for this to begin to normalize, and sometimes it never does. Fortunately, a fistula between the airway and the esophagus is rare, but you need to be aware of them, in case your child doesn't fit into one of the easier-to-deal-with causes of asthma and you are considering other diagnoses.

Also, I previously mentioned that an abnormally located artery in the chest can sometimes cause tracheal or bronchial compression and malacia. This malacia can persist.

I am wide open to parents getting their advice and medical interventions from a variety of different professionals, from the standard MD to Chinese herbalists, but as far as I know, no professionals other than pediatric pulmonologists and pediatric otolaryngologists and pediatric airway surgeons have much understanding of airway malacia. If therapeutic intervention is needed for airway malacia, it requires the experienced advice of one of these highly trained physicians.

CHAPTER 9

Your Child's Age and Asthma

Asthma symptoms are caused by different things at different ages (although with a *lot* of overlap). I have inserted this chapter here to help you to focus your thinking on what might be most relevant to your child. Unfamiliar terms in this chapter will be presented later.

Neonates (first month of life). If your newborn baby seems to have asthma symptoms at this age—including wheezing and difficulty breathing—I strongly urge you to converse with your doctor until you are satisfied that both you and your doctor understand the situation. Your doctor may see your baby and be quite sure things are okay and be able to reassure you. Or he might be concerned about your baby too and not be able to reassure you. There are many causes of airway narrowing and obstruction in small babies, and these need a lot of experience to sort out. Abnormal anatomy (things not formed the right way in a baby) can be a real problem and it needs to be considered. It may be as easy to deal with as a narrow nostril, or as severe as large arteries squeezing an airway, or *many, many* other things. This needs a conscientious doctor to help you decide whether it is appropriate to go see a subspecialist (a pediatric pulmonologist, most likely). Neonatal breathing problems are beyond the scope of this book. I cannot think of any neonate who should be diagnosed and treated as if they have some kind of routine "asthma." If your newborn baby has breathing problems, see a doctor right away.

Infants (first year of life). In many ways infants are similar to neonates when it comes to unusual things that can cause wheezing or difficulty breathing, such as anatomic abnormalities. But infants can also

51

have a lot of asthma symptoms caused by respiratory viral infections. Such children may be labeled as having "RAD" or Reactive Airway Disease. Chapters 14 and 15 are dedicated entirely to respiratory viral infections and RAD. *Viral bronchiolitis* is caused by respiratory viruses that infect and inflame the smaller airways in the chest (the bronchioles). In this age group, the *common cold viruses* can cause asthma exacerbations. Stuffy noses from viruses cause problems also.

Infants are not old enough to be allergic to inhaled allergens (such as dust and pollen), so allergic inflammation as a cause of asthma symptoms is uncommon in the first year of life (but remember, nothing is impossible, and every child is special). Reflux and aspiration (breathing in) of stomach acid and food can cause asthma symptoms. Malacia is a cause of asthma-like symptoms. Cystic fibrosis—now usually diagnosed with neonatal screening—can become apparent at this age (and is briefly discussed in a later chapter along with other, more challenging chronic causes of troublesome respiratory problems that sometimes can get confused with the more common causes of asthma).

Toddlers and preschoolers (age one to five). Viruses, including the common cold, trigger asthma symptoms in children this age who are prone to asthmatic responses. This *"viral-induced asthma"* is probably the most common type of asthma at this age. Inflammatory reactions to inhaled allergens (*allergic inflammatory asthma*) become gradually more important in causing asthma symptoms as these first years go by (but only in children who are allergic!). Previously unidentified anatomic abnormalities may rarely be an issue. Previously unidentified rare immunologic deficiencies and cystic fibrosis can show up now too.

School-age children (age five to teenager). Viral-induced asthma (on its own) becomes less common as the years pass. Allergic inflammation triggered by various allergens and *exacerbated* by the common cold becomes the more common cause of asthma in this age range. (This is *allergic inflammatory asthma*, with or without viral-triggering of asthma). If a child this age is not allergic, then the usual course is that her asthma will gradually go away over the years. If allergic, then the asthma sticks around through these years.

Because this chapter discusses age primarily, it makes sense to mention something that is important in allergic types of asthma. Children who are allergic *often* (but not always) follow a pattern of allergies and symptoms over time.

Here's the pattern. A baby may have eczema—dry itchy red skin caused by allergy to milk most commonly, or as he gets further into infancy, possibly an allergy to egg or maybe another food. Allergy testing can be done to find out. If your baby has allergic eczema (also called *atopic dermatitis*), you should know that it is quite common for her, as she is growing up, to develop allergic rhinitis (*hay fever*), and allergic asthma too, because of allergies to stuff she inhales (pollen, dander, dust). In other words, milk or egg allergy in babies with eczema is a precursor of allergic inflammation in the lungs, and asthma from that inflammation.

Actually, I often think of allergic inflammation in the airways to be "eczema of the lungs." The skin and the airways have a lot in common: they are two of the largest surfaces through which our bodies come in contact with our environment.

This is the time for another bit of confusion that I want to bring to your awareness, and then clear up. If a child has allergic inflammation as part of their asthma, the common cold viruses are usually big triggers of exacerbations of the asthma. Indeed, in children who have allergies to stuff they inhale, *the common cold* causes more trips to the emergency room and hospital than any other cause of asthma. Please recognize that there is *viral-induced asthma* in which the virus is acting without allergies to cause asthma, and there is *viral-triggered asthma,* in which the viruses do something to make allergic inflammatory asthma worse. These are two different, but probably related, entities.

CHAPTER 10

The Diagnostic Empiric Trial

You may be thinking now, "All right, I have learned about all these causes of airway narrowing and airway obstruction, but what is causing *my child's* asthma?"

I am *so* glad that you asked that question! Actually, I hope that by now you *have* asked this question, because if you *have* asked the question, then I know you have learned a most important lesson.

And that lesson is: *asthma is not a diagnosis, but rather a reason to go searching for a diagnosis.*

I hope you will excuse me for not (yet) addressing what is causing *your child's asthma.* But we'll get there. There are more tools to learn first.

Armed with the information in this book, you will be able to help your child's doctor find the diagnosis. Or potentially (and here's another trick) *several diagnoses* for your child's asthma.

It is quite common to have more than one cause of one child's asthma. One cause can be relevant at one time, and another at a later time. Or two or more problems can occur together, both leading to asthma symptoms. Just like viruses and bacterial infections and allergies and stress can all concurrently be relevant in *diarrhea*, multiple causes can be concurrent in *asthma* as well.

We'll go through the statistically likely contributors to your child's asthma over the next several chapters. The statistical likelihoods of the various causes of asthma are pretty well known. I know that your child is *not* a statistic. But the statistics are helpful as you and your doctor decide on the best processes to go through to seek your child's diagnosis and make initial choices (or initial *guesses*) for therapy.

A medical maxim is that "Common things happen commonly" and this is stated by doctors sometimes as "When you hear hoofbeats, expect horses, not zebras." It turns out that asthma in *school-age* children most commonly results from allergic inflammation in the airway. Thus, to doctors, *allergies* as a cause of asthma are the horses. But sometimes the asthma symptoms come from one of the causes mentioned earlier—some less common source of hoofbeats, and therefore referred to as zebras.

The current medical *system* focuses increasingly on treating the average person with "asthma" to optimize the average asthma outcomes in the population. That would be fine if we all had identical horses. But some children have zebras. In fact, pretty much all children have zebras at least part of the time. The groupthink average outcomes that the medical community has recently been taught to focus on don't serve well for those children, at least when they are galloping along with zebras. Because "asthma" is wrongly considered to be a diagnosis, the doctors are taught to think of asthma as all horses, and they don't often look to see if your child's symptoms happen to have black and white stripes.

Let's pause for a recap.

Asthma is recurrent episodes of reversible airflow limitation in the chest.

Airflow limitation can be caused by narrowing or obstruction.

Narrowing and obstruction can be caused by

1. Bronchospasm (from bronchial hyperreactivity/muscle twitchiness)
2. Swelling, including swelling from inflammation (of various different types)
3. Mucus and other material accumulating in the airways
4. Compression and/or kinking of the airways
5. Malacia
6. Congenitally small airways
7. Relative narrowing (greater than normal airflow going through normal or small airways)

Very commonly these processes overlap and contribute to each other.

Inflammation is a particularly important contributor to most of the other causes of narrowing and obstruction.

- Certain types of inflammation can lead to bronchial hyperreactivity (airway twitchiness) and bronchospasm.
- By definition, inflammation involves swelling, which also narrows airways. Inflammatory compounds also can turn on mucous gland secretion in the airways, as well as make it more difficult for the airways to clear mucus, and you already know that accumulating mucus is one of the potential causes of airflow obstruction.
- Inflammation is commonly associated with acidic pH as well, and acid can cause all sorts of injuries, and trigger bronchospasm and cough, and cause more inflammation and more mucus secretion.

Inflammation and acidification can be central to much of the underlying cause of airflow obstruction. We have no therapies for airway acidification *yet*, but we have lots of very good and safe therapies for *some* of the key components of airway *inflammation*. And because there are therapies for some types of inflammation, the doctors focus their asthma control efforts primarily on inflammation. That's understandable, and okay, because inflammation is important.

There does not have to be inflammation and/or acidification to have asthma. Inflammation underlies or at least plays an important role in *most* asthma in *most* children *much* of the time. We pay inflammation great attention. But inflammation is not universal, and, as mentioned before, inflammation comes in a variety of different forms, which do not all respond to the same therapy.

Is some sort of inflammation part of *your* child's asthma? That's the right question to ask. Statistically it is probable. But your child is not a statistic. How do we figure it out? Well, there are those two tests I mentioned in chapter 5—exhaled nitric oxide and sputum inflammatory-cell counts—that can measure inflammation, but you will be hard pressed to find doctors who have the setup to do those tests.

Also, there is an important type of test (which will be discussed in detail later), called *allergy testing*, that provides a bunch of information to your doctor that can help in many ways in asthma diagnosis and therapy. But allergy tests don't measure inflammation either; they assess the likelihood of having allergic inflammation.

Fortunately, there is another type of test, a *critically important* type of test, that is useful particularly in patients with asthma. It is a type of test that can be very helpful in optimizing the individual care for your child's asthma, and one that I hope you get very proficient at. It is a *wonderful* type of test for asthmatic children. In fact in many ways it is the best type of testing for asthma, and is perhaps the best way to figure out whether your child has certain types of inflammation (particularly allergic-type inflammation).

This test is called the "diagnostic empiric trial." In a diagnostic empiric trial, we give medication to your child and see how she responds. I want to discuss this at this stage so that you get used to the concept of "trying a medicine to see how it works" without concurrently thinking anything negative about the concept.

The diagnostic empiric trial is indeed a *test*. There, I said this twice, because it is important to not miss this point. People easily get confused about it because in a diagnostic empiric trial, we use one or more medications in your child to see if he gets better. We are not using the medication as therapy for the asthma. Not yet. Before we start *therapy,* we need to have a clue what is causing your child's asthma. Your child's response to the medications actually helps us to figure out what is causing her asthma.

For example, your doctor might start your child on inhaled steroids. If your child responds to inhaled steroid medications very well, and the asthma symptoms disappear, then that provides support for the concept that your child's asthma involves the destructive influence of a type of inflammation that responds to steroids—often this is allergic inflammation.

To try a medication and see how it works may sound a bit like trial and error, but it is actually a *great* diagnostic method to help figure out what type of asthma your child has. And a well-performed diagnostic empiric trial quickly can make a child who has had persistent asthma all better, quickly enough in fact to resolve our fears that there is something more troublesome in the airway. This can save discomfort and money that would have been unnecessarily spent on other diagnostic procedures. (Remember, *persistent* asthma is a cause for urgency in diagnosis, or a call to convert it — often using medications — to the more reassuring *intermittent* asthma.)

If your child doesn't respond to inhaled steroids, but instead responds to something altogether different, then we can suspect your child has an altogether different type of asthma.

The *diagnostic empiric trial methodology* not only helps diagnose underlying causes of asthma, but it also concurrently does something else of great importance. Right at the same time, it also determines if the therapy is one that might work well for *your* child. Because remember, even if your child has a type of asthma that most other children have, it doesn't *necessarily* mean that your child will respond to a medication the same way that most other children do. Children, every single one of them, are special and different from all the others.

Used correctly, the diagnostic empiric trial is a fantastic method to figure out what is going on in *your* child. It is a key part of *personalized medicine.*

Some tricks for diagnostic empiric trials of medications can be helpful to know.

First, I like to have some sort of objective measurements before starting an empiric trial. There are asthma-symptom rating scales that are simple to grade (they take a minute or two) that help to remind you how your child is doing initially. These go by various names, such as "Asthma Control

The other big parts of personalized medicine include (1) your doctor listening closely to you and your child; (2) your doctor being aware of non-disease issues in your child's life that impact the asthma and that asthma impacts; (3) other types of diagnostic and predictive tests; (4) careful tuning of interventions to your child's specific diagnosis and his special characteristics.

Test." Often these measurement questionnaires are designed to help pharmaceutical companies sell more of the drug that is most profitable to them, but they can still be useful. Your doctor probably has a preferred scoring system. The key thing is that it is a clinical score (meaning you can do the scoring yourself in a few minutes based on your child's symptoms).

Objective measurements of asthma physiology can be valuable to have before and after a diagnostic empiric trial. Lung-function testing (spirometry) can be performed in school-age children. This type of testing is discussed in the following chapter.

Then, with some gauge of your child's status before the diagnostic empiric trial, you start a medication, at the highest recommended dose, and see how it works over a period of time (hours to a month). The time should be sufficient both for the drug to work, and for you to have enough experience with it to see if it actually *is* working.

At the end of the trial period, you can do another asthma-symptom score test and your child can do lung-function measurements. You can compare the scores and lung functions before and after the diagnostic empiric trial, and then you will have knowledge about whether the drug works in *your* child. And that is much more valuable than knowing if the drug works in *other* children, isn't it?

It is true that an empiric diagnostic trial can lie to you, either because of a placebo effect, or because your child happened to get better (or worse) during the test period, entirely coincidentally, in a manner that had nothing to do with the test medication. But these lies sort themselves out over time. When things aren't true, they don't last for long.

When I am testing to see if a drug is going to make a patient's asthma symptoms better, I don't use a wimpy dose. I use a full dose, even what might be called a high dose. Why? Because if we start with a wimpy dose and don't get a response, then we will need to increase the dose and see what happens, and then increase further if still no response. Months can pass. To me that is silly.

So when I am performing a diagnostic empiric trial of a medication, I will prescribe a high but safe dosage regimen. If that medicine works, great! We then have very helpful information: specifically, that your child's asthma involves a pathway that the medication we tried actually helps to resolve. And then we can lower the dosage of that medication right down to the minimum right then and there, knowing that we may need to increase the dosage again, but with confidence that it *does* work in your child. If the empiric trial does not work, then we can put that therapy aside as unhelpful in your child's case (it might be wise to re-examine it later, because asthma changes). There will be no need to keep trying higher and higher doses, because we initially tried a high dose.

I perform these empiric trials with the benefit of a lot of experience. I don't recommend you try this on your own at home without the advice and guidance of your child's doctor .

High-dose inhaled steroid is a medication that I use in diagnostic empiric trials when I am seeking to determine if allergic inflammation is a cause of a child's asthma. Even "high dose" is really a tiny amount of inhaled medication compared to the swallowed oral steroids. A typical high dose of inhaled steroids for a school-age child might be 880 micrograms per day. At most, 20% of this is actually absorbed, so that is like 220 micrograms in the body. In comparison to the 40 milligrams of an oral steroid (like prednisone) that a school-age child would be given to treat an exacerbation of "asthma," this 220 micrograms is tiny. A microgram is 1/1,000 of a milligram. So the daily dose of high-dose inhaled steroids ends up being 181 times *less* steroid than *one* dose of the swallowed prednisone. It would take half a year of high-dose inhaled steroids to add up to one single modest dose of oral prednisone. But there is a caveat.

The inhaled steroids are more potent than prednisone, molecule for molecule. Because of that, perhaps a better estimate of the comparison is that about 30 days of inhalation of high-dose steroid is like one oral dose of steroid. It is all pretty rough estimation, but it helps give you a feel for the difference.

There are data that suggest that inhaled steroids do affect growth, but only very slightly. On average, that effect on growth is small. Indeed *final* height of children is not different based on whether or not they used inhaled steroids every day for years. But the fact that there is an effect at all makes me consider inhaled steroids to be not 100% safe. Like all medications, I want to use them if needed, but not when they aren't needed, and at the lowest possible long-term dosing. The first thing to do to help avoid unnecessary use of medication is to try to get the diagnosis correct.

CHAPTER 11

Lung Function and the Testing of It in Your Child

This chapter is focused on how your child's lung function is affected by asthma. It also will teach you the various ways doctors (and you) can assess lung function in your child at various ages.

Asthma is a physiologic disturbance, or an abnormality in the function of the airways. Thus, it makes sense that lung-function testing can help diagnose asthma and monitor it.

As you know, my definition of asthma includes *airflow limitation*. How have we identified airflow limitation so far in this book? I haven't talked much about actually measuring it.

The way that we know there is asthma is usually by the clinical finding of "wheezing" or noisy breathing, which is noisy *because* the airways are too narrow to allow air through them efficiently. Wheezing is the most commonly used indicator of airflow limitation and the most clinically valuable to you as a parent, too.

Doctors have other ways to identify airflow limitation too. For example, they (and you) can watch your child breathe. The worse the asthma is at the moment, the longer it takes to exhale. That is because the airways in the chest are squeezed closed a little tighter during exhalation (by laws of physics that I won't discuss in

Coughing is not an indicator of airflow limitation, but it is an important symptom that appears concurrently with airflow limitation in many types of asthma. In children who have asthma, coughing is a clue that airflow limitation might not be under control. Pay attention to coughing in your child with asthma.

this book), and stretched open a little during inhalation. The difference in airway size (caliber) between exhalation and inhalation causes the airflow limitation of asthma to be worse (and *usually* the wheezing to be worse) during exhalation than during inhalation. This causes it to take longer to exhale than to inhale. You can see this in your child if you watch her closely.

We've talked about airway narrowing as well as airway obstruction, both of which contribute to asthma. A narrowing means some air can get through. Complete obstruction stops air movement. In asthma, some or many airways close (obstruct) during exhalation when they should not. They may be inflamed, bronchospastic, or have mucus in them. But whatever the cause, when an airway is behaving this way, sometimes air goes *in* through the airway, but not all of it can get back *out* as the airway squeezes closed a bit more during exhalation. The air gets *trapped* in whatever portion of the lung tissue the airway feeds air to. After a while in which there are slightly more air molecules going *into* a part of the lung than are coming *out*, that part of the lung can get overfilled with air and stretched like a balloon.

In a child with active asthma, it is very common to have *air trapping* cause her lungs and chest to be overfilled with air. This *air trapping* causes the lungs to *hyperexpand.*

Please take a moment to try an experiment. It will help you understand asthma exacerbations. Take a regular, normal, small breath. In and out. It takes very little effort, right? Now fill your lungs really full with air, fill them to the brims, hold on to the breath, and then without exhaling first, *try to take an additional breath.* Try doing it now. That little bit of extra inhalation is *really* hard to accomplish, isn't it? It takes a lot of work.

In this little experiment, you have mimicked *air trapping.* Children with active airflow limitation may commonly trap air and can get enough air trapped in their lungs, with their chest stretched out so much, that it is hard to pull more air in. This causes children to work very hard to breathe and causes them distress. This distress and hard work of breathing is revealed by rapid breathing (*tachypnea* in medical parlance), as well as evidence of chest ribs and stomach muscles moving in and out hard and fast, and also anxiety.

When this is happening particularly badly, oxygen levels in the blood may start to decline, which leads to more anxiety, certainly, but is also an indicator of the need to get help quickly. Oxygen can be measured in the blood through a painless sensor on a fingertip called a pulse oximeter, which measures blood oxygen saturation and reports out a value as a percentage. You can buy one for your home very cheaply now.

What oxygen saturation is normal? Although there are some subtleties, a value between 95% and 100% is reassuring. To be clear, all that a normal oxygen saturation means is that oxygenation of the blood is okay. It does not mean that there is no asthma or other problem going on. But a nice oxygen saturation of 95% or more is reassuring that at least you have time to *deal* with any asthma that may be happening. A value below 92% is certainly concerning and requires intervention.

Of course if you are scared or think something isn't right, don't let a normal oxygen saturation by itself reassure you. Know your limitations and seek experienced help from a doctor.

Everyone knows that an increased breathing rate happens with lung

Fingertip oxygen-saturation testing (pulse oximetry) is easy to do at home, but there are tricks to it. You can buy a sensor on Amazon or at your local pharmacy for about $25 with no prescription. Read the instructions. You put it on your child's *warm* finger, make sure his arm and his hand are at rest and not wiggling (resting on a table or a pillow or a lap is fine). Then give the system a minute to figure out the oxygen saturation. It will show the oxygen saturation and the pulse rate on a little screen right there on the fingertip device.

These devices rarely report a falsely *high* result, but they can and frequently do report a falsely *low* value. So don't panic if you initially see a low number. There will be lights to indicate that the device is sensing the pulse in your child's finger. Those lights should be rising and falling with each heartbeat along a nice steady rhythm. If the pulse is *not* showing a steady rhythm, that usually means the device is not getting a good reading on the pulse, and it will report a false value. To avoid this, make sure your child holds still and is not wearing any sleeve or bracelet that is tight (and might lessen the pulse). Consider switching to a different finger. Also, it is wise to remove fingernail polish on the finger.

Monitoring your child's breathing rate (respiratory rate) can be helpful in tracking how his asthma is behaving. I recommend counting breaths while he is asleep (a good time is when you check on him before going to bed yourself). Count the number of breaths in a full minute. (*Don't* cheat and count for just 15 seconds and multiply by four!) Do this every night for a few nights when your child is fully healthy and sound asleep. The breathing rate should be similar each night—each night's measurement will probably be within 2-3 breaths/minute of the other nights'. This will be his *baseline, normal, sleeping respiratory rate.* Keep an eye on his sleeping respiratory rate in the future. If you count it almost every night when you check on him before going to bed yourself, it can give you a warning of impending problems with asthma. If it increases by 25%, trouble is probably brewing. Beware of catching him during restless or dream periods of sleep, when the breathing rate can be variable. You want to measure it when he is restfully sleeping.

disease. Increased respiratory rate is also a sign of disease in the airways that lead down *into* the lungs.

Beyond listening for wheezes (with your ear or a stethoscope), timing exhalation (how long it takes to exhale), and counting sleeping respiratory rate, there are formal ways of measuring lung function, most of which get done in a doctor's office (and if you get lucky, by professional respiratory therapists), but you can do some key ones at home as well, once you know what you are doing.

Formal lung-function testing is usually achievable if your child is 6 years old or older, and most often takes the form of *spirometry.* (There are other tests that we won't talk about in this book, and they are only available in clinics or hospitals staffed by respiratory therapists.)

Spirometry involves your child taking a very deep breath (the deepest he can take) and blowing out as hard as he can through a large tube until he empties his lungs as completely as he can. A device measures the volume and the flow rate of air that comes out. There is no pain involved, nor danger, and it tells us a lot about airflow limitation.

Performing spirometry correctly is important, or it can be misleading. The need to do it correctly is why it is not commonly performed under the age of about age 6 years old. (I have seen children as young as 4 years old accomplish it, though.) There are even *infant* lung-function tests, but they involve sedation and are not commonly performed.

Here are the key tricks to performing spirometry correctly. Remember this is for *school-age* children.

1. Your child must seal his lips around the tube that will measure his breath. This tube is not a straw, but *much* bigger, about an inch in diameter.

2. Your child must first take the deepest breath possible. He must fill his lungs to the very tippy top (and do this *every* time he does a spirometry test). This is the most essential step.

3. When the respiratory therapist performing the tests says "Blow!" your child needs to blow as hard as he can for as long as he can without stopping, and keep blowing even when it feels like there is not another molecule of air left to come out (which may be just a few seconds of blowing, by the way). Keep blowing until the respiratory therapist says to "breathe in" again, or to "stop."

It is really easy to blow out for a long time through a tight straw, and indeed a tight straw is kind of what your child will be expecting from years of shooting spitballs. *But*, a straw is *not* what your child will be blowing through during spirometry. Rather it is a much bigger tube that offers no resistance. Without resistance, it is hard to keep blowing when

---

The lung has ways to help send blood flow to segments of the lung that are getting fresh air into them (oxygen) and to *not* send blood to parts of the lung in which the airways are obstructed. This system, called *ventilation-perfusion matching*, is constantly adjusting the blood flow in each segment of the lung to match how much oxygen is filling the lung sacs. This very cool system keeps as much blood as possible going only to areas of the lung that are moving air normally. This keeps your blood supply optimally oxygenated, even when there are areas of the lung that aren't working at all. Because of this, however, your child can have normal blood oxygen saturation in the presence of airways that are obstructed from active asthma.

The lung system that maintains this good blood oxygenation only works to a certain point. When too many airways are obstructed, the system fails. Also, some of the medications we use to treat bronchospasm can interfere with this system of balancing blood flow and airflow in the lungs. For this reason, we don't want to use a medication if it isn't helping.

all the air gets out really fast through that wide tube.

Indeed, children with no airflow obstruction can finish their exhalation of air within 2–3 seconds, and won't be able to get any more air out after that no matter how hard they push. But children with airflow narrowing can blow for longer, because it takes more time for the air to come out through the narrowed airways in their chest, rather like they are indeed exhaling through lots of tiny straws. Because of this, it can be more comfortable for children with airway narrowing to do spirometry than for healthy children to do it, although children with active asthma may cough during spirometry. In children with severe airflow limitation (asthmatic or other), it can take 10 seconds or more to finish exhaling.

The longer exhalation time in a child with airflow limitation is not because they are exhaling more air, but because they are exhaling it more slowly (even though during spirometry they are pushing as hard as they can to blow it out). The better his lung function is, the faster a child can blow out his air.

There is something else to clarify. Children (and adults) do not really empty their lungs when they blow "all their air out" of them. Actually there is a lot of air left in the lungs that cannot come out. The amount of air that cannot come out tends to be larger during active asthma than when healthy. This is that *air trapping* mentioned earlier. When asthma is severe, the air trapping can be pretty big.

Spirometry usually is performed three times in a row to make sure the test is accurate. It provides several pieces of information, right away, about lung and airway function.

Forced Expired Volume in 1 second (FEV1). This is the most commonly helpful measurement. It is the volume of air that your child can get out of his lungs in the first second of forced exhalation. Starting from a completely full inhaled breath, the FEV1 is the measure of how much air he can force out, when he is pushing out as hard as he can, in the first second. It is a pretty good measurement of airway narrowing. Children with active asthma tend have lower FEV1 than when they are healthy. This makes sense, because children with active asthma may take 8–15 seconds to exhale their air, so less of it will be in that first second of effort.

Forced Vital Capacity (FVC). This is the total amount of air that your child can blow out, starting from a completely full inspiration, blowing out hard, until his lungs are as empty as he can get them. Children with active asthma may have normal or low FVC compared to when they are healthy.

Peak Expiratory Flow (PEF). This is also called *Peak Flow,* and is measurement of flow, not volume. It measures the fastest speed that your child exhales any time during her effort at forced exhalation. A low PEF is considered a marker for large airway narrowing (such as in the larynx or trachea), but it is also low when there is narrowing in the bronchi and below in smaller airways. The Peak Flow can be readily measured at home and in the past was used a lot in asthma management, but is used less often now. I rarely ever use it in management of patients, but the use of it was part of standardized asthma guidelines for so long, and the test pushed by the National Institutes of Health in all sorts of programs, that many doctors still rely on it. It does have value in some situations.

Forced Expiratory Flow between 25% and 75% of exhaled volume (FEF25–75). This is sometimes called "midflows" and is a measurement of the average flow rate during the middle of your child's forced exhalation maneuver. When FEF25–75 is low, it suggests smaller airways are narrowed (down below the mainstem bronchi). This value is the most sensitive to asthma, meaning it will usually start to fall first as your child's asthma starts to worsen at the beginning of an episode of an asthma exacerbation.

These values and others from spirometry help physicians quantify your child's physiologic airway narrowing and obstruction at the time of the test. This can then be compared over time to help quantify effects of treatments focused on improving asthma.

For home, you can buy an inexpensive device that you can use to measure PEF, FEV1, and something called FEV6, which is the volume of air a child can exhale in the first six seconds of forced blowing. It is not the same as FVC, except in healthy children with no airway or lung disease. But the FEV1 can be helpful. Just do an Internet search for "home spirometry" and you will find some choices.

In summary, at home, you can recognize the presence of airflow limitation by listening for wheezing, monitoring sleeping respiratory rate, watching your child breathe, or performing tests with an inexpensive ($50) home spirometer. And you can measure oxygen saturation at home too with the additional $25 spent on a pulse oximeter.

The spirometer that your doctor has will do a more precise and complete job of assessing your child's lung function than one you can buy. But spirometry only reports the lung function at the time of the testing. Asthma can increase or decrease a lot during even one day. Both home assessment and professional assessment of lung function therefore makes sense. If you and your child get good at home lung-function testing, you will have a lot more knowledge and power over your child's asthma.

Testing for bronchial hyperreactivity (BHR) is performed in a lung function laboratory at specialty clinics. This test involves performing spirometry before and after inhaling something that is known to promote bronchospasm in people who have twitchy airways. It might be dry air, or a compound called methacholine, or a concentrated salt solution, or a sugar called mannitol. Any of these can be used to determine how twitchy a child's airways are at the time of testing. We don't do these tests often, because they take a lot of time. But knowing if BHR is present or not can be helpful when trying to sort among all the causes of what is often diagnosed as *asthma*. Such testing can also help show how well a course of therapy is working. It is unlikely that your child will undergo this testing outside of university hospitals at this juncture.

Exercise can also be used as a challenge to determine bronchial hyperreactivity.

You and your doctor, knowledgeably working together with your child and complemented by various objective lung function tests, will arrive at the best methods to keep asthma quiet.

CHAPTER 12

Radiographic Studies

This is a sweetly short chapter that provides information about x-rays and other similar studies that are performed for asthma diagnostic purposes.

When a child presents (appears) with asthma symptoms for the first time, it could certainly be one of the common causes of asthma (a horse), but it could also be a less common cause (a zebra). When a child first has asthma, we won't be certain what the diagnosis for the asthma symptoms is.

Given that there are occasional zebras that cause wheezing and asthma symptoms, and some of those zebras are important to know about early, I usually obtain an x-ray of the chest the first time a child wheezes, pretty much regardless of age. The first time your child wheezes, I will want to make sure there is nothing funny going on in the chest—no pneumonias, nothing that seems likely to be kinking the chest airways, no areas of collapsed lung, and a normal heart shape on the x-ray.

Later on, once a reasonably confident diagnosis (or diagnoses) for your child's asthma has been established and you know what you are dealing with, obtaining x-rays with each wheezing episode is rarely helpful. But occasional x-rays of the chest may be warranted if things change. Each child is different, and her asthma can change.

A CT scan of the chest is only occasionally needed. CT scans are 3-dimensional x-rays. I sometimes use CT scans to examine the chests of children whose asthma is not making sense, if the symptoms don't add up right, or the response to therapy is not as I might expect. A CT scan can give me information that an x-ray can't.

Nuclear scintigraphy (nuclear-medicine studies) can be helpful in identifying if a child is aspirating food or fluids into her lungs during swallowing, or refluxing and aspirating, both of which might guide me toward treating stomach reflux as a cause of asthma. It is a bit tricky because such a study only examines one episode of eating, and can miss reflux and aspiration that only happens now and again, so I rarely use these studies.

For most children, an initial chest x-ray is all the radiographic investigation that I use in diagnosing and managing asthma.

That is why this chapter is short! In fact, this is the last sentence of this chapter!

CHAPTER 13

Allergies, Allergy Testing, and Allergic Inflammatory Asthma

Allergies play a dominant role in *most school-age* children with asthma, and in many *preschool* children. They only rarely play a role in an infant with asthma symptoms.

If your child has allergies, your child's immune system is misbehaving. Don't be fearful about there being some sort of really bad immune deficiency. That's unlikely (but not impossible... see chapter 21 on *confounding diagnoses*). Allergies that are relevant to asthma are a pain in the butt, but usually are not dangerous.

I will try to present the vast amount of information that doctors know about airway allergies all within one digestible chapter.

A child can develop an allergy to food, or to small inhaled particles, or to medications. These allergies share a certain type of immunologic process that can happen within minutes of an exposure in a child who has been previously *sensitized*. A child can also develop contact sensitivities to things that touch his skin, such as poison ivy and certain metals, but these are a different type of immune process that is usually slow (days after exposure).

For asthmatic children, the most important things that cause allergic problems are the small inhaled particles that float around in the air or cling to pillows.

Things that trigger allergic reactions are called *allergens.* The most relevant allergens are listed here:

- Pollen
- Pet Dander
- Dust
- Molds

Most allergens are proteins (as opposed to carbohydrates or fats).

When it comes to asthma, it is *inhalant allergens* that are the most relevant ones. Inhalant allergens consist of microscopic particles your child inhales.

The most common inhalant allergen in most home environments (and also the most common thing to be allergic to in general) is *house dust mite*. Dust mite is a major contributor to house dust (but not to industrial dust in factories). Dust mites are little bugs that are too small to even recognize without a microscope. They are a bit smaller than the period at the end of this sentence. Dust mites aren't cute. Figure 3 shows what they look like.

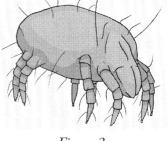

Figure 3

Dust mites live in your child's pillows and mattress. There can be millions of the little buggers in our bedding. They don't bite you or your child, so don't worry about that. In fact, if your child is *not* allergic to dust mites, they'll cause him *no harm at all*. They are just one of the many critters we share our planet with. However, if your child *is* allergic to dust mite, it is commonly a source of lots of trouble.

Dust mites walk through the stuffing in our pillows and mattresses like we walk through air. Their favorite source of nutrition is the dry bits of skin that flake off us all the time.

> Did you know that another major component of house dust is human skin flakes? Yuk! But don't make too big a deal of it. We've lived a long time with dust, and it's mostly okay.

Where do most skin flakes accumulate? In our mattresses and pillows while we are sleeping. That's why dust mites like to live there. Dust mites eat our flaked off dry skin bits, digest them, have little dust mite babies every couple of weeks, and, as all critters do, poop. It is the microscopically tiny bits of dust mite poop that actually contain the proteins to which children can develop allergy.

Dust mite poop particles are just the right size to easily breathe into our nose and mouth. If they were much bigger, they wouldn't lift into or be carried far in the air. If they were smaller, we might breathe them in and then right back out again like a gas molecule, and they couldn't cause any problem. But dust mite poop particles are just the right size for children (and adults) to inhale into their nose and lungs, and for the particles to get trapped in our airways where they just might interact badly with the immune system.

Again, if your child isn't allergic to the dust mite poop, it won't cause her a problem. The airway has good systems for clearing out any tiny particles your child inhales that land in her airway. One of the normal jobs of mucus is actually to help your airway clear out such trapped particles.

But if your child has developed an allergy to dust mite, then dust mite poop particles in the nose or lungs can trigger allergic inflammation including swelling and bronchospasm and mucus production and acidification and accumulation of immune cells—you know, all those things that we know cause narrowing and obstruction.

Pollens (from grass, trees, and weeds) and pet dander (cats, dogs, rabbits, guinea pigs), feathers, and molds (both indoor and outdoor molds) can all behave very similarly to dust mite allergens if they get in the nose or lungs of allergic children. In fact, these allergens I just mentioned are the most common inhaled allergens.

Let's take a break for a moment to remember something: allergies are very common in children who have asthma symptoms, but not every child with asthma has allergies.

Does your child have allergies that may be triggering or worsening her asthma?

We can find out.

I start by asking if there is a family history of allergies. Does Mom or Dad or a sibling have any allergic diseases? Allergic diseases that I consider important are:

The skin, eyes, nose, lungs, and gut (intestines) are the parts of the body that most show the evidence of allergic reactions. This is because these are the parts of the body that interact with the environment most directly and come into contact with allergens directly. These body parts are populated with cells that contribute to allergic inflammation.

- Some types of asthma
- Some types of eczema (dry inflamed skin)
- Allergic rhinitis (hay fever), and/or allergic conjunctivitis (allergic eyes)
- A history of recurrent "bronchitis" (because bronchitis is a term sometimes given for asthma)

If there is no family history of these illnesses at all, the chance that your child has allergies is substantially lower than average.

But, really, if your child has asthma, then your doctor will likely be suspicious of allergies regardless of family history, and will probably want to find out directly whether *your* child is allergic. And that can be done with special testing that is easy to obtain.

Allergy Testing

There are two common types of allergy testing: skin tests and blood tests.

Skin tests measure the presence of the allergy antibody, called IgE, that is *attached to mast cells in the skin*. There can be IgE that binds to cat dander, or IgE that binds to dust mite, or to any of lots of other allergens.

Blood tests measure these same IgE antibodies that are floating around *free in the blood*, as opposed to attached to cells.

Both types of tests look for IgE antibody .

Skin Tests

Skin tests are usually done in the office of an allergist, which means a visit to that specialist. Allergists specialize in knowing all about the topic of allergy and are also experts in many types of asthma. Some children may see an allergist just once during their diagnostic process for asthma. Others may be partially managed by an allergist working alongside your child's pediatrician or family practitioner, or even entirely managed by the allergist. There are no rules about this. We should all choose whatever makes sense.

Skin tests are not just testing for *skin* allergies. Testing the allergic response in the skin is a pretty effective way of testing for how the *nose and lungs* will respond to the same allergens. Allergic sensitization (being allergic) is not localized to just the lungs or just the skin. It is a whole-body thing, which allows us to test the skin and use that to help us understand the lung.

Skin testing is usually performed with "skin pricks." These are not painful, and your child will not suffer any pain with them at all. There is nothing to fear.

> IgE is an antibody. The IgE molecules are supposed to recognize parasites, but in the modern day, the IgE sometimes foolishly recognizes and binds onto allergens. Remember, allergens should cause us no harm on their own: pollen is harmless, left to its own devices. It is actually the foolish IgE that causes harm by binding onto the poor allergen!

That there is "nothing to fear" does not mean your child will not *be* fearful, depending on his age and how much fear you as a parent and we as doctors might unintentionally suggest they should have. One of the most fearful things a parent can say to a child on the way to a doctor or before a procedure is "There is nothing to be scared of. It won't hurt a bit." The combination of the child's ears and brain commonly end up with him only hearing the words "scared" and "hurt."

It's best not to say anything other than "We will learn a lot at the allergist's office to help you feel better and stay healthy."

Skin tests involve taking a tiny droplet of an allergen in liquid out of a bottle and pricking it into the very top level of your child's skin with a tiny device. It is small and so superficial that is feels like, at most, a single tiny hair pull. The allergist or her nurse will probably do multiple tests for different allergens all at the same time.

These skin pricks are done on the non-hairy parts of the inner forearm, occasionally on the upper arm, or on the back. Your child may get tested for six allergens, or he may be tested for thirty allergens. The number of skin pricks will be the same as the number of allergens being tested for, plus two. The two spares are *control* tests.

Antihistamines need to be avoided for up to a week or more before the date of the skin testing. Antihistamines are medications that block the effects of histamine, and accurate interpretation of allergy skin tests depends on histamine functioning normally. So no antihistamines before the skin tests! (Follow the allergist's instructions that they will provide before you come to your child's appointment).

A *negative control* shows how your child's skin will respond to just the effects of the prick, without allergen, and consists of a liquid with no allergen in it. The *positive control* is usually *histamine*. Histamine causes a certain type of allergic response that causes inflammation. This is used to see how your child might respond to the actual allergens pricked into the skin. Occasionally an allergist might do a third control test.

I want to take a moment to make sure you know that your child cannot have taken any antihistamines for a period of time before the skin tests are done. Antihistamine treatment will mess up the allergy skin-prick tests. Different allergists have different rules about when the last dose of antihistamine is allowed to be taken. Also, the number of days your child needs to be "antihistamine-free" before skin testing is different for the different antihistamines.

Antihistamines are used to treat allergies, the common cold, vertigo, and to prevent car sickness and nausea. Any medication you buy that is designed to treat those illnesses might have in it an antihistamine that could foul up the allergy skin tests.

There are dozens of antihistamines on the market. They have different names in different countries. Below is an alphabetical list of antihistamines that is adapted from the work of the helpful folk of Wikipedia (and used under Creative Commons attribution http://creativecommons.org/licenses/by-sa/3.0/).

I have put the most common antihistamines used in the United States and their US names in *italics*. If you are in another country, the brand names are likely different. Examine the list for the generic drug names and compare them to your child's medications.

List of Antihistamines

- Acrivastine
- Azelastine (Astelin nasal spray)
- Bilastine
- *Brompheniramine (Dimetapp)*
- Buclizine
- Bromodiphenhydramine
- Carbinoxamine
- *Cetirizine (Zyrtec)*
- Chlorpromazine (Thorazine—an antipsychotic)
- Cyclizine
- *Chlorpheniramine (Coricidin, Rynatan)*
- Chlorodiphenhydramine
- Clemastine (Tavist)
- *Cyproheptadine (Periactin. Also used for migraine prevention and to stimulate appetite.)*
- *Desloratadine (Clarinex)*
- Dexbrompheniramine
- Dexchlorpheniramine
- *Dimenhydrinate (the original Dramamine) (most commonly used for car sickness)*
- Dimetindene
- *Diphenhydramine (Benadryl)*
- *Doxylamine (Nyquil)*
- Ebastine
- Embramine
- *Fexofenadine (Allegra)*
- *Hydroxyzine (Vistaril)*
- *Levocetirizine (Xyzal)*
- *Loratadine (Claritin)*
- *Meclizine (Bonine) (most commonly used for car sickness or to treat vertigo)*
- Mirtazapine

Generic drug names are generally not the same as *brand* names. For example, one well-known antihistamine goes by the brand name "Benadryl," but the generic name is diphenhydramine. Diphenhydramine is the ingredient in Benadryl, and it is also in a bunch of other over-the-counter medications sold to treat allergies and colds.

- Olopatadine (Patanol eye drops)
- Orphenadrine
- Phenindamine
- Pheniramine
- Phenyltoloxamine
- *Promethazine (Phenergan—an anti-nausea drug)*
- Pyrilamine
- Quetiapine (antipsychotic; trade name Seroquel)
- Rupatadine
- Tripelennamine
- Triprolidine

Some allergists will also ask your child to not take certain types of stomach-acid-blocking medications, because these can also somewhat interfere with some histamine responses. These include

- Cimetidine (Tagamet)
- *Famotidine (Pepcid and Pepcid AC)*
- Lafutidine (not available in the US)
- Nizatidine (Axid)
- *Ranitidine (Zantac)*
- Roxatidine (not available in the US)

If your allergist asks you to avoid these before skin-testing day, make sure to ask for how long avoidance is needed. Note that *proton pump inhibitors*, another major class of stomach-acid-blocking medications, do not interfere with histamine at all and can be taken before allergy testing.

Do be aware that most of the over-the-counter cold medications contain an antihistamine. Look on the list of ingredients. There are dozens of brands of cold medications for sale in the United States, but they are all various combinations of 1, 2, or 3 drugs chosen from just a tiny handful of medications. Actually, most of them are pretty much the same as the others. Read the labels to see if there is an antihistamine in a medication before giving it to your child before skin-test day.

As a final caveat, if your child *needs* an antihistamine badly (such as to treat a big allergic reaction or to prevent car sickness), it is probably okay to reschedule the skin tests, or ask the doctor to do blood allergy tests instead (which are *not* affected by antihistamines).

The allergy skin tests take about 10–15 minutes (after pricking) to show up before they are read (interpreted). During that time, your child must not scratch them. And *that* is a challenge, because the histamine (positive control test) will cause itchiness, and any allergens pricked into his skin to which he is sensitized (allergic) may well itch also. But he *must not scratch*, because scratching will mess up the tests. Also, we don't want the liquid containing the allergen from one skin-prick site to be accidentally wiped into another prick site, because that would confuse any skin responses that appear. So, don't let your child even touch the skin-test sites until the skin tests have been read by the nurse or doctor performing them. It is okay to blow across them though, and that can be soothing as well as distracting. Speaking of distracting, it is great to read a book, or watch a video, or sing songs during the testing period.

What should you expect from the skin testing? Well, after ten minutes or so, the positive control (histamine) prick should look like a mosquito bite—raised, red, itchy. This is like a small hive. And the negative control should look pretty much like normal skin. We'll get to what the allergen pricks may look like in a moment.

If the histamine (positive control test) doesn't look like a mosquito bite, the whole panel of tests becomes questionable. It may be that your child indeed did take some antihistamine that you forgot about or didn't know (such as at school). Remember, antihistamines mess up the test. It is also possible that the positive-control histamine didn't prick well into the skin and a repeat of just the control may be reasonable to try.

If the negative-control (no allergen) test looks like a mosquito bite, then also, the whole panel of tests becomes questionable. Some children have skin that indeed does respond by getting a hive (a red itchy bump) *whenever* their skin is scratched or pricked with *anything at all*. Such children have *dermatographism*. You can actually write on their skin with a fingernail because, a few minutes later, the skin swells up and turns red just underneath wherever it is scratched. Dermatographism is created by hives, and goes away in half an hour or so. Anyhow, if the negative control looks like a positive, then we really cannot trust this set of tests this time, can we?

Fortunately, most of the time, the positive control will be positive and the negative control will be negative. And if the skin tests do happen to fail, it is okay to try blood tests.

Okay, back to the allergens. If your child is sensitized to an allergen, the skin test should look like a mosquito bite. Raised, red, and itchy. If there is a very strong allergic response, it can look like a *big* mosquito bite with a strange shape with legs like a fat starfish. The size of the response gets measured by the nurse or doctor, and may be from a couple of millimeters to as big as an inch if there is a major allergic sensitization. Mostly, an allergic sensitization will show in a skin test that is a few millimeters in size (less than a quarter of an inch). If your child is not sensitized to a given allergen, the skin at that prick site will be flat.

The nurse or doctor will read the skin tests and interpret them and then they will tell you what your child is allergically sensitized to. We'll get back to the results in a little bit.

But first, some allergists may also perform intradermal allergy skin tests. Not many allergists do intradermal testing in children for inhalant allergens, but some do. These tests involve needles injecting little pockets of liquid into the skin. They are performed just like a PPD (the skin test for tuberculosis), except that the PPD is read in 48 hours, and the intradermal allergy test is read in 10–15 minutes. Intradermal tests are a little more risky, can be more painful, and children don't like them much. They are often used to assess drug allergies, but there are debates as to whether they add value in the evaluation of inhalant allergies in children. They may have more value in complicated evaluations in adults, though. Your allergist can guide you. I can tell you that it would be a very rare child indeed on whom I would use intradermal allergy tests when evaluating asthma. But every child is different, and doctor's experiences are different, and the fact that I don't use them much does not mean that they aren't a good tool for other doctors.

How about Allergy Blood Tests?

Allergy tests can be done by drawing a tube of blood from your child's arm and sending it off to the laboratory. The blood tests measure IgE (the allergy antibody) floating in the blood. It can take from one to five days to get the results back, so the doctor won't be able to counsel you about your child's allergies then and there like they can with skin-testing results. Blood tests work fine even if your child has taken antihistamines lately.

Any doctor can order the allergy blood tests, but allergists are much more experienced than other doctors in interpreting blood allergy test results. Blood-test results for allergies can be overinterpreted if the only thing that the doctor does is read the lab report. You see, there may be mild elevations in the IgE antibody in blood that are entirely irrelevant to your child's asthma. The interpreting physician needs to know allergies well, asthma well, and your child and the environment in which she lives.

What Do I Learn from Allergy Testing That Will Help My Child?

Another great question! Once you find out *what* your child is allergic to, what do you make of that information? We will have a chapter on "environmental control of the home" soon.

But for now, here are some useful generalities.

Your doctor most likely will test your child for many of the common *indoor allergens* as well as *outdoor allergens*. There are different reasons to test for indoor allergens and outdoor allergens, but they share one reason that makes it worthwhile to test for them: if your child is allergic to *any* inhalant allergen (or to most food allergens as a small child), it proves that your child is an *atopic person*, which basically means that he is an allergic person and is inclined to allergic responses. In regards to asthma, the main thing about being *an atopic person* is that the asthma is likely to have an *allergic inflammatory component*, and the allergic inflammation of the airways is usually treatable in ways that other types of inflammation are not. So, when I see a school-age child with asthma, it is important to know if he is atopic (allergic) because it helps me hone in on the *diagnosis* of *allergic airway inflammation* as a cause of his asthma, and to focus empiric trials on this allergic inflammation, leading to more rapid and complete improvement in your child's health.

We'll discuss indoor allergens first.

Indoor allergens include: dust mite (two species of them), cat dander, dog dander, cockroach, and sometimes common indoor molds. Also, if warranted by your child's environment, the doctor may test for guinea pig, bird feathers, or whatever sort of pet your child might have. Or your doctor may test for mouse or rat, if your child is exposed to such creatures. Other irritating pests that sometimes plague houses and that can cause allergies include Asian lady beetles — and, soon enough, I expect, stink bugs.

The indoor allergens share, in general, the notion that you can *control* your child's exposure by lessening the amount of allergen around. Now, those of you whose homes are infested with Asian lady beetles or stink bugs may be howling with pained laughter at some doctor's foolish notion that those damn things can be controlled. I know. I've been there.

But how about dust mites, cat and dog dander, or cockroaches? Your child's exposure to these allergens *can* be controlled, with effort. And in the chapter on environmental control, I will discuss some of this.

Remember, a main purpose of testing for *indoor* allergens is to determine if there might be value to putting effort into controlling the amount of allergen around, because less allergen often means a healthier child.

In that regard, a lesson I want you to learn now is that if your child is *not* allergic to a given allergen, you don't need to go to effort to control the exposure. The so-called "allergens" are indeed *not* "allergens" to *your* child unless your child is actually allergically sensitized to them, as proven by skin or blood tests. "Allergens" don't cause your child harm, not at all, *unless* she is allergic to them.

One exception (there are always exceptions, aren't there?): when there is a high likelihood of your child developing allergies in the future, or *more* allergies over time, your doctor might recommend not getting a cat as a pet. New allergic sensitizations can develop over time in people who have an allergic nature and an allergic family. And cats might well become trouble for allergic children. So it is best to not invite in the trouble of a new cat if your doctor thinks there is a reasonably high risk of allergy developing.

Outdoor allergens that allergists test for include geographically appropriate tree pollens, grass pollens, and weed pollens, as well as molds.

Allergists in each part of the country and world know what people are most commonly allergic to in their region, and what outdoor allergens are most worthwhile to test for. This is true even if you are moving around from one region to another or from one country to another.

It is pretty much impossible as well as unnecessary to test for every plant that pollinates to see if your child might be allergic to it. There are too many. And molds, wow! There are zillions of them. And it actually doesn't help much for you to know *exactly* what species of plants or outdoor molds your child might be allergic to.

Here's why:

You can't do a thing about them.

If you live in Virginia, and find that your child is allergic to the pollen of a certain tree, what can you do—chop down all the trees of that species between Virginia and the Mississippi River? That pollen blows on the wind all over the place! The pollen particles are microscopic and carried by the air from your neighbor's yard, the park down the street, and the golf course three counties over. There's nothing you can do to stop that pollen.

So now I will add something confusing. Data show that if children are not allergic to cat, then living with a cat may *prevent* them from developing an allergy. Whoa, what did I say? If this is the case, then why do I recommend *not* getting a cat? Because, first, *your child* is not "children," nor is he "data." And the words "*may* prevent" are not "*will* prevent." The trouble with getting a cat for someone who is a generally allergic person (allergic to other things) is that allergy to the cat "may" *eventually* develop. And by the time it does, the cat is loved and can't get removed without great heartache and most likely will stay around inciting allergic inflammation in your child's lungs. Having a cat in the house of a child who is allergic to cats and has asthma can be real trouble! Sometimes it is better to avoid the heartache.

But, although you can't stop the pollen from flying around, it is counterproductive and silly to live in fear of pollen or to keep your child in an indoor bubble (please don't!).

Yet it *is* helpful to know whether or not your child is allergic to the pollens of trees, grasses, and weeds, as well as the molds that are all floating around outside. Why? Because with the knowledge, you can be aware of *when* your child might have worsening allergic asthma, and intervene *in advance*.

You see, trees and grass and weeds pollinate during specific seasons and specific months. In the mid-Atlantic states in the United States, for example, trees pollinate in the early to mid spring, and grasses pollinate in May and June; weeds pollinate starting in late August through the autumn.

If your child has asthma symptoms, and if you have noted the asthma to be much worse in the months that grass pollinates where you live, and if she is found on testing to be allergic to grass pollen, then bingo, you have identified a likely *diagnosis* for her asthma: *asthma from allergic airway inflammation triggered by grass-pollen sensitivity.*

That's the first example of a fully complete asthma *diagnosis* that I have given you. It includes the cause: *allergic sensitivity to grass pollen*; the type of inflammation: *allergic inflammation*; and the symptomatic and physiologic result: *asthma*.

Ahh, now *that* is a *diagnosis*.

And that diagnosis is *very* different and needs different therapy than other diagnoses that cause asthma, including:

- Asthma from allergic airway inflammation triggered by *dust mite* sensitivity
- Respiratory-virus triggered asthma
- Exercise-induced asthma
- Stomach acid reflux–induced asthma
- And many others that we will discuss in the next several chapters.
- And, importantly, combinations of these various causes of asthma.

I have to caution that it is very common for a child to have several interacting causes of his asthma, which means more than one *diagnosis*.

If your child has the diagnosis of "asthma from allergic inflammation triggered by grass pollen sensitivity," you are well armed with key information that will help guide therapy and get the asthma under control. You know the cause of your child's asthma (or one of the causes at least), you know in what months the asthma will likely flare (the months that grass pollinates), and you know that it is likely to be allergic inflammation underlying the asthma, and we can teach you what generally works to treat allergic inflammation. That's a lot of knowledge to guide you. And it is much more helpful than being diagnosed with "asthma" and having drugs thrown at you according to some protocol written by doctors somewhere near Washington, DC.

You see, with this diagnosis in hand, you can move on to best help your child, using any of a variety of means.

You might start anti-allergy medications in your child a week before the grass starts to pollinate, including, for example, starting inhaled steroids and maybe nasal steroids, montelukast, and maybe antihistamines. There will be more information in this book on these drugs. But for now, know that *preventing* impending airway inflammation is an easier task than treating established inflammation, so it can be very helpful to start the medications *before* the pollen even gets in your child's lungs.

You might start your child on regular allergy shots, or allergy drops under the tongue, to desensitize your child's immune system to grass pollen. These are done through allergists, and not all allergists offer this *allergy immunotherapy* for the treatment of asthma. In some countries, allergy immunotherapy is not recommended for asthma at all. But, as you might guess, I like it when you work with your doctor to make individual decisions to help your child, as opposed to relying on some national recommendation.

Did I mention that your child might have more than one diagnosis underlying her asthma? Oh, yeah, I did.... And you will want to know all of your child's diagnoses. Keep reading.

I do not recommend keeping your child inside during allergy seasons. Children should play!

Knowing that your child has grass-pollen allergy will allow you to be aware of the higher risk of asthma exacerbation (worsening) in the grass-pollen months.

The same holds true if your child is allergic to "weeds" or tree pollen, but just shift your months of medication and wariness around slightly.

I am reminded to mention another important tidbit: *allergy season* is a groupthink term. The so-called "allergy season" usually means spring and fall. But *allergy season* may differ for each child. Because you and I are focused on *your* child, you should be asking, "What is *my* child's *allergy season*?" That's a great question and one that can be answered by having allergy skin tests or blood tests performed. Your allergist can then tell you when the stuff your child is allergic to is going to start floating around the environment each year.

It may be that your child is allergic to trees, grasses, *and* weeds, and therefore spring and fall are filled with pollens that trigger allergic airway inflammation that causes asthma in your child. Let's pretend this is the case. Then the diagnosis your child has could be *asthma from allergic airway inflammation from sensitization to tree, grass, and weed pollens.*

Or, your child could be allergic both to the outdoor allergens (trees, grass, weeds, and mold), *and* the indoor allergens such as dust mites and cats. Indoor allergens are generally perennial (year round), as opposed to seasonal. If your child is allergic to all sorts of things, both indoor and outdoor, it may be simpler to skip naming the specific inciting allergens, and diagnose it as *asthma from allergic airway inflammation from indoor and outdoor allergens.* This is okay shorthand. But *you* should know the details of the allergies, because when it comes to the indoor environment, you can have some control over your child's exposures.

Treatment for the diagnosis *asthma from allergic airway inflammation from sensitization to indoor allergens* involves not only medications, but also, to the extent possible, control of your child's exposure to these indoor allergens. (Remember, the indoor allergens are dust mite, cat and dog dander, and some molds, cockroaches, and the less common pet exposures or pests.)

There is a chapter on environment control coming up in a bit.

A note on allergy testing in infants. Infants (first year of life) haven't had time to develop allergies to pollens or indoor allergens. The earliest I have seen an allergic-test response to an inhalant allergen was in a 9 month old, and that was to cat (a very potent allergen). Usually inhalant allergies don't appear until about 2–3 years of age.

But infants can be allergic to foods they eat. Milk, soy, egg are the most common allergens at this age, but other foods an infant eats might also occasionally cause allergies.

Skin tests for the foods can be performed in infants after a few months of age, and food allergies can be relevant to asthma in infancy. Allergy testing in infants can prove a child is *atopic* (meaning he has an allergic tendency) and this can help you and your doctor anticipate what may be coming in the future.

The term *allergic inflammatory asthma* is what I will mostly use in this book as a *diagnosis* for the type of asthma in children with inhalant allergies. It is not as specific a diagnostic term as *asthma from allergic airway inflammation from sensitization to grass pollen,* but it is nonetheless specific enough for us to make wise decisions about therapeutic choices for your child. The term *allergic inflammatory asthma* is convenient and sensible and pretty precise.

CHAPTER 14

Respiratory Viruses: The Common Cold and Others

The common cold is a royal pain in the arse. When you are sick with it, you can be miserable, it pretty much ruins a week, and on top of that, it generates hardly any sympathy from others, but rather turns you into a temporary pariah. And we have no treatment for the common cold that seems to work worth a darn.

Sure, there are lots of cold medications available over the counter. They treat some of the symptoms of a cold, but if you have tried them you have probably discovered that they don't do all that much other than make you sleep. The reality is that they provide *some* symptomatic relief in *some* people. What about children? Well, almost all the big studies say that cold medications not only don't work to treat colds in children, but they may even cause a little bit of harm. In preschool-age children, that risk can be bigger, and infants bigger still. Most general pediatricians will advise you not to use cold medications.

My recommendation? Well, every child is different, and your child wasn't enrolled in one of those big studies, so it's not like you *know* these cold medications *don't* work in your child. But these cold medications have no reason to work *much*, and *certainly* won't cure a cold, and if they do help in your child, they probably won't help much. In infants, I suggest just skipping them altogether. In preschoolers, I think chicken soup is the best medicine for colds.

In the school-age child, you can either skip the cold meds, *or* give them a try to see if they seem to make *your* child better. If the effect in your child is not enough to be sure of, then it isn't worth giving. If the effect is very clearly beneficial, then use it, and try it again with perhaps a bit of reasonable cynicism during the next cold and see if it works then too. It may not. Or it might. Try it and see. It's an empiric trial.

Oh, the cold medications will not in any way prevent an asthma exacerbation.

Most of the cold medicines—despite all the different brand names—are just combinations of a small handful of drugs: usually a pain medicine (either acetaminophen or ibuprofen), a decongestant (pseudoephedrine or phenylephrine), and possibly an antihistamine (one of several). The antihistamines that are included in these cold preparations are usually of the older class of *sedating antihistamines*, and not the new non-sedating antihistamines, because the most valuable perceived effects of antihistamines in the treatment of a cold result from their side effects.

Although histamine plays a real role in allergies, it plays but a small role in the common cold. Blocking histamine with antihistamines therefore doesn't do much good to treat colds. But the older antihistamines have side effects that include sedation (which helps you sleep through a cold) and something called "anti-cholinergic" properties. The anti-cholinergic properties may provide a bit of symptomatic relief in a cold, sometimes helping to dry a runny nose, maybe.

One comment about decongestants. These are used to open stuffy noses, and they actually do work in a lot of kids (not all). As cold medicines they are given orally, but other types can be sprayed up the nose. They work by causing blood vessels that are overly widened to shrink, and to cause normal-size blood vessels to narrow. They squeeze blood vessels. Part of a congested nose is from widened (dilated) blood vessels. In fact it is dilated blood vessels and the blood flow in them that causes inflamed tissue to be red (*rubor*—the first Latin word in that good old definition of inflammation). The dilated widened blood vessels also tend to leak clear fluid out of the blood, which makes the tissue of the nose more congested and wet. And they provide fluid for the glands in the nose to excrete, which makes noses more drippy. So a decongestant can provide some symptom relief for a cold by countering these things. But they can also cause blood pressure to rise (from squeezing blood vessels everywhere in the body) and speed up the heart rate, and there are other risks, and for those reasons often pediatricians recommend against using them.

But, every child is different. I find that in some small children who have particularly bad malacia, a stuffy nose from a cold can cause them such great distress that they may need hospitalization, sometimes even in an ICU. All from a stuffy nose! Although pediatricians and family practice doctors are now taught to not use decongestants to treat the common cold in children, it is important to remember that there are times when these drugs can be useful. Decongesting the nose in a child with airway malacia can be one of those times. It is a trick to be considered after the diagnoses in your child are established reasonably confidently, and with your doctor's awareness and approval.

It is always worth reinforcing that antibiotics do nothing to treat a cold. Antibiotics treat bacteria, not cold viruses. Please don't pressure your child's doctor for antibiotics to treat your child's cold. Antibiotics are not at all risk free. They may well even increase the risk of asthma. Use them when needed, and not when not needed.

In a child prone to asthma, the common cold can be much worse than a pain in the arse. During preschool years, the common cold can cause asthma exacerbations and this can happen frequently—several times a year or more. Remember, the cold medications do *nothing* to prevent asthma from happening. If your child has allergies and asthma, then during the school-age years, the common cold may repeatedly trigger asthma exacerbations in him. Indeed, the common cold is responsible for the asthma exacerbations that cause most asthma hospitalizations and most asthma emergency room visits.

I mentioned several times now that our *treatments* for the common cold are pretty poor and ineffective in most children. The only *prevention* is to avoid getting infected.

It seems to me that there are endemic cold viruses in every town and city, and that these circulate around and infect every new member of the community, especially the children. In addition to getting sick with colds, children are also *viral vectors*, which means they are little reservoirs of the common cold. A surprisingly large percentage of healthy children with no cold symptoms carry the common cold viruses up their noses, ready to infect somebody who comes along on whom a child wipes a booger or two either directly (such as while crying) or through objects that he has touched.

In different towns and cities there may be different endemic viruses. Now and again, the cold viruses pop over to other towns and cities and cause little cold epidemics in them. It turns out these annual cold epidemics in North America most commonly happen in April and September. Who knows why? Summer vacation and spring break, maybe? When trips to other places happen? Perhaps. Maybe the viruses just like going on road trips.

When a cold virus to which the child has not before been exposed infects him (usually through rubbing the germ into his eyes, nose, or maybe his mouth), a cold commonly (but not always) results. Children get a lot of colds during the first few years that they are exposed to other children. In prior generations, the exposure to other children usually began in earnest at age 5 or so, with the start of school. Nowadays it starts as soon as daycare begins. So kids get all those colds starting at much younger ages.

Your child may be in daycare, or may not be. Whether your child is (or was) in daycare or not is one of the factors that, along with many others, contribute to the uniqueness of your child and your child's asthma.

A young child in daycare with other children tends to catch the colds that the other children keep up their noses. Those other children catch the colds your child keeps up his nose too, so, tit-for-tat. Absent a tendency to asthma, or airway-narrowing disorders like malacia or chronic lung diseases, most little children do just fine with all those colds they pick up in daycare, other than being a bit fussy and maybe getting some bacterial infections (like ear infections) as an after-effect.

If your infant or preschool child is one of those children who does *not* tolerate colds well, who gets malacia symptoms or asthma symptoms with a cold—then it is wise to try to protect your child from getting colds until he is older and bigger. The airways get bigger as your child gets bigger; the airway cartilage gets firmer too. The bigger the airways are, and the firmer the cartilage is, the fewer problems will arise from the effects of a stuffy nose.

Colds stink for some children as infants, and for some children when older.

Realities of parents' jobs make daycare hard to avoid for many people. Here's my recommendation: if possible, try to avoid daycare if your infant or preschool child has clearly shown lots of troubles with breathing when he gets colds. (Note: avoiding daycare is rarely a *mandatory* thing—it is really only mandatory in children with very severe airway disease.) When your child gets even a year or so older, he may tolerate those colds better. Your doctor can help you sort it out.

Now's a great time to remember that I probably have not been introduced to your child either. I am therefore one of those "experts who hasn't met your child." Your child's doctor is your best advisor when it comes to your child's asthma. This book just helps you be the best partner to your child's doctor in sorting it all out and figuring out the best ways to control the asthma.

The summary is that the common cold (and other respiratory viruses) cause asthma-like symptoms in preschool children prone to asthma. And cold viruses also trigger asthma exacerbations in school-age children with inhalant allergies.

A Word about Influenza

Influenza is bad sort of virus that rears its head every winter in North America. Influenza is not the "stomach flu." It's a totally different thing.

Please don't be paranoid about respiratory viruses. Once you know about asthma, it is almost always manageable. The more you know, the easier it is to deal with asthma. It does require patience, sure, but the odds are excellent that your child will, in the long run, do well with asthma. Keeping a child in a "bubble" in the hopes of avoiding infection isn't a great idea. Keeping your child perfectly clean and germ-free is possibly even a bad idea because your child does need to develop immunities to the infections in the world and thus needs some exposure to them, and it seems that natural social interaction provides that exposure pretty well. Also, although we aren't really sure, we have reason to believe that children with less exposure to germs have a higher risk of allergies and asthma a bit later. That's under debate right now, but at least suggests that dirt and germs aren't all bad. There is a good side to almost everything!

Influenza causes high fevers, exhaustion, body aches, nasal and lung congestion, and a horrible cough (and it can cause vomiting too). Influenza tends to be particularly tough on some (maybe most) children with asthma. We don't yet know which types of asthma are most adversely impacted by infection with the flu, but we do know that on average, kids who get asthma symptoms tend to get them worse when they get influenza, and are more likely to be hospitalized than children who don't get asthma symptoms. Influenza is something to avoid if at all possible.

Children over age 6 months and most adults can get vaccinated each fall for the strains of influenza that experts guess are going to be the strains that spread around the most. Most years the professionals guess pretty well.

There are several different flu vaccinations available by injection, as well as a nasal flu vaccine (squirted up the nose). As of this writing, the nasal vaccination is not recommended in children with recent wheezing (within the last year) because of, actually, an increased risk of wheezing, so for now, let's stick with the injected version for most asthmatics, because the injected form does not increase risk of wheezing. But please note that the nasal-spray version is actually preferred (and more effective than the shot) for most other *non-asthmatic* preschool and school-age children.

The first year that a child gets influenza vaccine, he should get two doses, one month apart. After that, it is one shot (or nasal squirt for nonasthmatics over age 2 years) every fall.

There is a low-grade chronic fear flowing through the Internet that vaccines are dangerous. So far, we have no way to know if a vaccine is actually going to be dangerous for any *individual* child. Until we do know how to tell, we have little choice but to rely on statistics, which are fortunately very good statistics, to guide what we should do for our individual children regarding vaccinations. And the statistics show that significant problems from most vaccines (including influenza vaccine) are exceedingly rare. Overall each individual child is much, much, much more likely to be *protected* by vaccines from a horrible complication of a bad disease than they are of suffering something horrible *from* the vaccine.

Measles is a horrible disease, as is mumps, as is meningitis, as is diphtheria, as is tetanus, as are hepatitis A and B. We can now, through science, prevent children from suffering from these diseases that have ravaged lives for ages. Horrible diseases, or diseases that cause real trouble for people with certain diseases (such as influenza can cause for people with asthma), are worthy targets for vaccines.

Based on my interpretation of the literature, here is *my general* recommendation about influenza vaccinations in particular. If you have a child with asthma, I recommend everyone in the household over age 6 months (barring contraindications to the vaccination) be vaccinated for influenza each fall to help prevent the virus from getting into the household and, in turn, protect the asthmatic child from the danger that influenza poses.

Every child is different, of course, and the decisions regarding childhood vaccinations can only be made by parents. I do recommend some humility in regard to the knowledge upon which you make your decision. Beware of Internet information as your sole resource. Lies and misinformation are promulgated in all forums at every level of society, and I have seen more lies about vaccines on the Internet than other places. Most vaccines are not developed for nefarious purposes. Most vaccines truly help much more than they hurt. I do have reservations about some newer vaccines, but I don't have any reservations about the flu vaccine for families of asthmatic children.

CHAPTER 15

Reactive Airway Disease

There is a disease entity referred to as Reactive Airways Disease (RAD). Doctors all over the world use the term, and because it is such a big issue among children with asthma, you need to understand RAD. I will try to help with that in this chapter.

Infants and preschool-age children (i.e., *young children*) get described as having "Reactive Airway Disease" or RAD if they have lots of troubles with intermittent wheezing and coughing and difficulty breathing, and if cold viruses trigger these troublesome symptoms in the chest instead of the cold staying up in the nose and throat where it is supposed to stay.

RAD is a term that, like *asthma*, is not really a diagnosis. RAD is a label given to infants and preschool children who basically have the symptoms of asthma, but are too young for a doctor to want to label a child as "asthmatic."

RAD is a term used for the various types of asthma that occur in infants and preschoolers when there is a reasonable possibility of the child outgrowing the problem. A good percentage of children with RAD will indeed no longer have troubles with RAD symptoms after several years have gone by. Those that persist with intermittent RAD symptoms throughout childhood will at some point get labeled "asthmatic."

From my viewpoint, if an infant or preschool child has episodes of airflow limitation in the chest (as evidenced by wheezing, junky noises, and hard work of breathing), and these go away and come back repeatedly (reversible and recurrent), then that child clearly has some illness that is causing him to have *asthma*, but in small children this situation is called RAD by most doctors.

A doctor might say to you, "You're child *might* have asthma, but we don't know yet, so for now we just call it RAD."

If your child has RAD, your next question of course should be "What is causing my child's RAD?" Right? Because RAD is not a diagnosis any more than asthma is a diagnosis

Let's look at an infant *without* RAD for a moment. An infant *without* RAD will catch colds (viral respiratory infections) in daycare, and the colds will cause a runny and stuffy nose, irritability, and maybe ear infections, but almost all the symptoms stay up in the head, not in the chest.

In contrast, when a child *with* RAD catches a cold, he'll get swelling and mucus production not only in his nose, but also in the airways of his *chest*. A child with RAD will wheeze and cough with colds, have junky noises in the lungs, breathing difficulty, poor eating, retractions (seeing the ribs when breathing), and sometimes a child with RAD will need a trip to the emergency room.

Why do some infants and small children have the misfortune of having RAD? Fair question. There is no certain answer, but I will tell you some of my thinking.

Remember, in my book (and this *is* my book after all!) RAD is just a term for asthma in infants and preschool children. And of course asthma has multiple causes. So does RAD.

Let's go through a few different ways that RAD occurs. Keep in mind that any one child could have one or more of these causes of RAD.

First, in an infant (whether or not the child has RAD), a stuffy nose causes the child to work harder to move air through her nose. Now, if she has *floppy* airways (whether formally diagnosed with *malacia* or not), the extra workload of a stuffy nose causes her to use her chest and abdominal muscles both to *suck air in* and *push air back out* of her lungs through that narrowed nasal airway. This sucking in and pushing out with every breath distorts the airways a little. The floppy airways in the chest flop with every breath, and make noise. The flopping back and forth stresses out the airway tissue, and it can get a little sore and a little inflamed as a result. It's kind of like a flag blowing in a wind; the flag can fray just a little as it whips back and forth; or it is like rubbing at an itch on your skin too hard: if you do it too much, the skin gets inflamed and weeps fluid and hurts. The same effects can happen in the thin walls of airways. The repeated strain on the airways can lead to inflammatory swelling (narrowing). Also, glands respond by secreting more goo (causing obstruction), bronchial muscle gets more twitchy, and the asthma symptoms ensue from the narrowing and obstruction. All of this started by just a stuffy nose in children with floppier airways.

> The anatomy of the very young infant simply does not allow breathing through her mouth, even when the nose is very congested. Neonates and young infants are *obligate nasal breathers*, and they will struggle to breathe if both nostrils are obstructed.

RAD from floppy airways is often a mild but frequent issue. The floppy airways show up at least a little bit even when the child does not have a cold (see the earlier chapter on malacia). These children are noisy breathers whenever they are excited or angry or sad, but get even noisier when they get the common cold. Such children often get lumped into the term RAD, even though the various causes underlying RAD are remarkably different from each other.

Here's another way RAD can happen. A fever causes a child to have to move much more air in and out of the lungs to satisfy metabolic needs for oxygen. In a small child with *narrower-*(smaller-) than-average airways, the airflow through the airways of the chest can get more turbulent (and therefore more noisy) when children have to move more air, and the turbulence causes airflow to both press against, and suck on, the cells of the walls of the airway in strange ways, like little tornadoes scooting along the airway walls. The cells of the airway aren't supposed to be exposed to this irregular pressure and suction (the suction can be like micro-hickies). Inflammatory swelling, glandular secretion and bronchospasm can result, leading to asthma symptoms. (Note that some turbulence can be good, for example by helping inhaled particles get trapped in the secretions on the walls of the larger airways before being carried far down into the lungs. But *abnormal* turbulence is not a friend). See Figure 4.

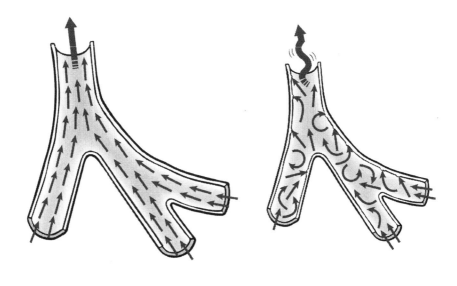

Normal airway with laminar flow   Smaller airway with turbulence

Figure 4

RAD that results from smaller-than-normal airways is hard to diagnose. In fact, unless the airways formed very wrong in a child, we don't diagnose "narrow airways" with any confidence. But sometimes a doctor might say to a parent of a child with RAD, "Your child's airways are narrow and that is why he is sick a lot, but he will outgrow it." Although the doctor isn't really sure of the cause, he is very probably right that the child will outgrow it.

Turbulent airflow. Optimally, air should flow through a child's airway smoothly, flowing along pretty nice straight lines all in parallel. This sort of flow is called *laminar*, and it is a quiet sort of gentle breeze through the airways that you can hardly hear. If, however, there is a narrowed airway with a lot of air trying to get through it, the airflow loses its nice straight line of flow and starts swirling around instead, bouncing off the walls of the airway and making the walls shake and vibrate. This sort of airflow is called *turbulent* flow. Turbulent airflow is *noisy* (wheezy, whistly, rough) and it also takes a lot more breathing energy to move the air when it is flowing turbulently. Narrowed airways mean more turbulence.

Here's the next (and entirely different) way I think RAD happens that isn't just in children with smaller and floppier airways. It will take the next several paragraphs to explain, so I will put a nice subheading here to separate it out. Indeed this subheading is also because this next way that RAD happens is a *very common cause* for asthma in infancy and preschool years.

Viral-Induced Asthma

There is a respiratory viral infection called RSV, which stands for Respiratory Syncytial Virus. RSV is a pretty bad virus that infects the lower airways (in the chest) of infants and causes an acute viral lung disease that is generally called *bronchiolitis* (meaning inflammation of the bronchioles) but the more appropriate term is "RSV bronchiolitis" or "viral bronchiolitis." Almost every child will catch RSV (from some little friend or other) within the first year or two of life. Some get bronchiolitis from RSV, and some just seem to have a bad cold with it. Some children get RSV more than once, but usually the first episode is the worst.

Children who get RSV bronchiolitis bad enough to come to the attention of doctors (as opposed to staying home) tend to be either (1) sicker with it, or (2) smaller/younger when they first get it. Those children who do come to medical attention (because they are sicker) commonly have more asthmatic respiratory problems throughout their childhood.

Asthma associated with early RSV infection goes away as children get older and is gone before teen years. But that doesn't mean that *asthma* necessarily goes away. If a child later *also develops allergies* to stuff they inhale, like dust mite, then she can develop an altogether different type of asthma, such as "asthma from allergic inflammation from sensitization to dust mite," which is a form of *allergic inflammatory asthma*. Allergic inflammatory asthma, unlike asthma after RSV, usually persists. Allergic inflammatory asthma can overlap in time with the asthma

Viral-induced asthma and allergic inflammatory asthma are entirely different diseases that are each pretty common and that show up with similar symptoms (asthma symptoms!).

initiated by the RSV. It can certainly get confused with the RSV-initiated asthma. They are two very different diseases however.

Whether there is any cause-and-effect relationship between RSV asthma and allergic asthma is not known.

Small children who had a bad episode of RSV tend to get asthma exacerbations whenever they subsequently catch a common cold. During the first few years of life, this tendency to have asthma exacerbations with colds gets lumped into the semi-diagnostic term "RAD" (although it is but one of many different causes of RAD).

For children in their infancy and preschool-age years who repeatedly get asthma symptoms when they get a cold or respiratory virus, I prefer the term *viral-induced asthma* instead of the term RAD. Viral-induced asthma is not a perfect term. But it is more precise than "RAD." Indeed, "Viral-induced asthma" is almost a diagnosis. It's not perfectly descriptive, but it is much more precise a term than "asthma."

If a child does not have allergies (based on skin or blood testing), then the viral-induced asthma may be the only type of asthma in that child, and the asthma will almost always go away as he gets older. But if he also has allergies, than I recommend watching for "allergic inflammatory asthma" as well.

The term *viral-induced asthma* is an appropriate term for young non-allergic children who get asthmatic with colds. "Induced" means "initiated by." In this case, RSV may initiate changes in the airway nerves and glands and other airway cells, and this makes the airways in these children particularly sensitive to getting asthma symptoms when a cold infects the child's *nose* later. Why can RSV do this? We aren't sure. I have a potential explanation, but it is pretty science-heavy, and mostly theoretical, and you can skip it if you want.

Here it is.

We know that RSV infection *increases* a type of sensory nerve in the airways that senses acid. This nerve type also senses heat and a chemical called capsaicin. Capsaicin is the stuff that makes hot peppers taste "hot."

This nerve sensor was evolutionarily designed in mammals to detect heat and acid, and to protect us from them. The pepper plant just took advantage of it to prevent mammals from eating it (that didn't work with humans! Yum!). You see, the pepper plant wants to spread its seeds through the digestive tract of birds, which, unlike mammals, can't digest and destroy the seeds. Birds have no nerve sensor for acid/heat/pepper, so birds can chow down on the peppers, which makes the peppers happy as the birds fly around and drop the undigested seeds along with some fine fertilizing guano into the awaiting soil. Or into my eye.

You know how your nose runs when you eat hot peppers? That is because these nerves in the mouth cause glands to secrete fluids in your nose.

These heat/acid-sensing nerves aren't just in the mouth, but also in the esophagus and in the lungs. When triggered by heat or acid (or peppers for that matter), these nerves send signals to the central nervous system and to other areas of the lung. These signals trigger reflex responses, including (1) cough, (2) bronchospasm, (3) glandular secretion in the lungs, and (4) cellular inflammation. In other words, they cause the stuff that underlies the physiologic disturbance you and I call "asthma."

There is evidence that the lungs get acidic during common cold infections, even in healthy people who don't get asthma. So if RSV infection has caused an increased sensitivity to acid by turning on lots of these acid/heat/pepper-sensing nerves in the lungs, and a child later gets a cold, the airway acid that occurs with the cold can cause an asthma exacerbation.

The good news is that over years, those acid-sensing nerves (that RSV caused to increase in number), gradually disappear down to a normal level. And therefore these children "outgrow" their viral-induced asthma.

So, respiratory viruses can cause stuffy noses that lead to RAD/asthma in children with floppier airways. They can cause fevers that lead to RAD/asthma in children with narrower airways, and they can lead to RAD/asthma in children whose airways were adversely affected by a bad or early RSV infection. As I mentioned, this last type of RAD — *viral-induced asthma* — is the most common.

Respiratory viruses may cause trouble for your child by causing asthma symptoms through any one of these mechanisms described

Ah, now it might make sense to you why hot peppers "burn" your mouth even though they aren't at a high temperature. Or why acid is said to "burn" even though it is not hot. You see, these nerves sense heat, acid, and peppers all the same way, and so these nerves cannot tell them all apart. To your nerves, heat feels just like acid and just like peppers.

It is important to know that just because your child has "asthma" doesn't mean he will have it forever. Indeed, viral-induced asthma is commonly outgrown. The type of asthma that children tend to have "forever" is the "allergic inflammatory asthma." There are a lot of those children. But even those children can almost always be so well managed that their troubles with asthma barely affect their lives, their activities, or anything else.

above, or combinations of them all. It is a pain in the butt until it goes away, but, unless your child is allergic, you can take comfort that asthma caused by viruses usually does go away long before age 13.

Oh, by the way, viral-induced asthma is a pain in the butt because it makes our little ones sick and miserable. It is also a pain in the butt because many "anti-asthma" medications really don't work well when asthma is caused by small or floppy airways, nor do they effectively treat either the original RSV-bronchiolitis, or the subsequent viral-induced asthma episodes. Our asthma drugs work great for asthma from allergic inflammation, but not for viral-induced asthma. It is no fun as either a parent or a doctor feeling powerless to make a child feel better. Yet that is how I feel frequently with viral-induced asthma. I do have some tricks for it, though, and I will tell you them in the chapters on therapy (coming soon!).

I will mention one other condition here, because it fits. *Post-bronchiolitis cough syndrome* is the name used to describe infants who get bronchiolitis (usually RSV), recover from it, and then cough for as long as four months. What a very frustrating thing! I speculate that the cause of this is exactly what I described above, with those acid-sensing nerves being too hyperactive, and very possibly with some stomach acid reflux then setting them off to cause cough and inflammation. But we don't know for sure.

Summary: Reactive Airway Disease (RAD) is a term I don't love. I prefer to try to decide what type of asthma it really is. Airway malacia is a diagnosis itself and conspires with a stuffy nose as one cause of a child's RAD. *Viral-induced asthma* is the term I prefer for non-allergic (or not-yet-allergic) children without obvious malacia in whom colds cause repeated episodes of asthma. In most cases, it is tough to prevent the acute episodes. But fortunately this type of asthma tends to go away on its own as the years go by. I will talk about treatment for these types of asthma a little bit later in the book.

Shaking hands with people is polite and friendly, and passes the common cold all over the place. During viral epidemics, it would be very wise for us to adopt the Japanese bow for the sake of avoiding the handshake....

CHAPTER 16

Stomach Reflux and Asthma

If in your child the common cold triggers asthma episodes because of airway acidity, and if this acidity causes overly acid-sensitive nerves to trigger an asthma flare, then you can easily imagine that *any* acid that gets into the airway might cause asthma flares.

One source of acid that gets into the lungs is *chlorine gas* from swimming pools. Chlorine gas gets inhaled and acidifies the airway. The airways in most children deal with that acid well, and neutralize it. Some other children may be particularly sensitive to chlorine, either because their airways can't neutralize the acid fast enough, or because their airways have too many acid-sensing nerves; in either event the nerves will trigger inflammation, mucus secretion, bronchospasm, and cough (just as I suspect happens after RSV infection in some children).

For now, just be on the lookout to see if your child seems to have trouble with chlorine and pools, especially indoor pools. If your child has no trouble, then don't worry about it. Swimming is a great sport for *most* children who have asthma!

We pulmonologists are often suspicious about another source of acid that can get into the lungs. *Stomach acid* can reflux up the esophagus (swallowing tube) and trickle over the larynx, through the vocal cords, and get aspirated (sucked down) into the trachea. See Figure 5.

For years, we recommended swimming as great exercise for asthmatic children because the wet air can help in asthma. But we have to remember that every child is different. Some children do poorly with chlorine in early life but do fine later. In others, the opposite is true. Love your child, pay attention, don't be paranoid, and certainly don't jump to restrict your child's great opportunity for fun in pools!

109

The larynx is very well designed to prevent food from getting into the airway during swallowing. There is a complex nerve and muscle interplay that assures it successfully does its job when your child swallows. The larynx is ready to close, just the way it should, as one begins to swallow.

But when food is coming back *up* the esophagus from the stomach in the opposite direction than usual, then the larynx doesn't know it's coming; it is not prepared to close, and only knows to close when some food or acid actually lands inside of it. And that is just a tad bit too late, because the stuff has already got down in the airway. So reflux from the stomach up the esophagus is much more likely to get into the airway than is food that is swallowed.

In other words, the larynx protects the airway very well during swallowing, but not so well during reflux.

Some children reflux more than others. Some children tolerate reflux and acid aspiration without symptoms. In other children, reflux and acid aspiration causes asthma and other respiratory problems, either because they aspirate a lot, their airways cannot neutralize the acid well, or because there are too many acid-sensing nerves.

In the medical community, we don't really have our heads around the relationship between acid reflux and asthma. It is a source of much debate. There are conflicting data about how much stomach acid reflux and aspiration into the airway is relevant to asthma.

What I can tell you with unequivocal certainty is that in *some* children, acid reflux plays a big role in their asthma.

We doctors, and you too, must remember to think of each child as an individual, and consider acid reflux and test for it when it seems appropriate; sometimes testing with acid-measurement techniques, but more often with diagnostic empiric trials of stomach-acid-blocking medications, to see if acid reflux might be causing some or much of your child's asthma. Acid reflux is not the first or most likely cause of asthma symptoms. It is one of many causes, and may be very minor in most people, yet a major cause in some. Which is it in your child? You and your doctor will need to be thoughtful, conscientious, caring, and even

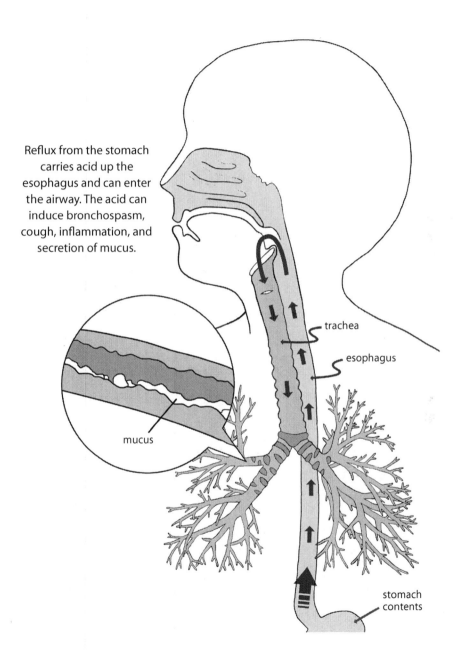

Reflux from the stomach carries acid up the esophagus and can enter the airway. The acid can induce bronchospasm, cough, inflammation, and secretion of mucus.

mucus

trachea

esophagus

stomach contents

Figure 5

patient, to figure it out over time. We'll discuss this more in the chapters on therapy.

It is clear from research studies that it does not make sense to treat *all* asthmatic children to block acid reflux. The problem with the groupthink in our medical system currently is reflected by the insurance companies, which, because of such studies, now often refuse to pay for acid-blocking medicine for treatment of asthma in *any* child, as if it doesn't work. But the data that insurance companies rely on (to refuse payments) lump all asthma together (even though there are many different types of asthma). Such data do not apply *at all* when you have a child who has acid reflux *causing* his asthma. In such a child, stomach-acid-blocking medications work very well indeed.

The only thing those studies say is that it doesn't make sense to treat *all* asthmatics with acid blockade. But it makes an abundant amount of sense to treat *your* child with acid blockade if stomach acid is causing his asthma, don't you think?

By the way, children reflux stomach acid a lot more when they are having trouble breathing. So even when reflux is not a problem when the airways and lungs are fine, the reflux may happen when your child is sick: when her asthma is exacerbating. That's an unfair double whammy. It can happen in infants and older children.

You see, a child can get an asthma exacerbation from a virus or allergic exposure, and start coughing and wheezing and have difficulty breathing. With time and medications, the virus will clear, the inflammation will go away, and the asthma symptoms will resolve, *except* if the trouble breathing also increases reflux, which it can do, and then the child can aspirate small amounts of stomach acid into her airways, and that aspirated acid keeps the asthma going for a long time, like picking a scab or rubbing a rash. We need to know about reflux and consider it. Reflux may not happen in most children most of the time, but it certainly happens in some children some of the time.

By the way, that reflux exists in a baby is most commonly pretty obvious. If your baby burps up after he feeds (wet burps), then he refluxes. No special zillion-dollar tests are needed to prove that a baby refluxes when you sit there and watch him burp up milk all over your shoulder! Most babies reflux. If he is a wet-burpy baby and he has lots of wheezing, then stomach acid reflux might well be a factor.

Also, even without acid, refluxed stuff can be aspirated into the airways. Milk and other food material can cause inflammatory responses in the airway.

Speaking of inhaling milk, we should also keep in mind that a baby may conceivably develop asthma symptoms if she is allergic to cow's milk and she inhales it into her airway (even little drops of it now and again). She could develop *allergic* inflammation in her airways (quite similar to inhalant allergy inflammation in older children). Allergy testing can find milk allergy in a baby. Sometimes it is necessary to change a baby's milk or infant formula because of lung disease.

CHAPTER 17

Exercise-Induced Asthma

Exercise is a common trigger of asthmatic responses. By this, I mean that exercise is a common trigger of *recurrent episodes of reversible airflow limitation in the chest.*

Your child doesn't have to be allergic, and he doesn't have to have inflamed airways, for asthma to occur with exercise, but allergies that result in inflamed airways certainly increase the chance that exercise will trigger asthma.

Whoa. Let's stop right there for a moment, because I don't want you thinking for a second that your child's asthma will always limit her exercise, nor that you should plan to limit her physical activity. Appropriately diagnosed and treated asthma should almost never inhibit your child's ability to play any sport, as aggressively as she sees fit, most of the time. It is a goal of appropriate diagnosis and therapy of asthma to make sure that exercise asthma is controlled/prevented/blocked/ treated as much as is needed to make sure your child's asthma is nearly irrelevant when it comes to athletics.

You have all heard stories about famous elite athletes with asthma. They are true. Once the diagnoses and therapy have been given full consideration, it is uncommon for asthma to significantly limit a child, other than for brief periods.

It is very wise to *not* have your child overexert himself when *he is in the midst* of an active asthma exacerbation (such as a viral-induced asthma episode or an allergic inflammatory asthma episode). Overexertion can and does worsen an already-occurring asthma exacerbation. It can even be dangerous. But you almost always can get your child to a point that her asthma is under such great control (so few exacerbations) that it doesn't interfere with any of her athletic dreams.

115

So please don't jump to limiting your child's activities. Instead, focus the effort on assuring your child's asthma does *not* limit his activities.

Alrighty then; with that point made clear, let's talk about why exercise triggers asthma.

When a child runs (or whatever type of exercise is undertaken), she will usually breathe through her nose initially. She will be able to breathe through her nose until the need for oxygen increases because the muscles are using up the supplies already available in the blood. It is difficult to move the air into the lungs fast enough when breathing through the narrow passages of the *nose*, so after a few minutes of exertion, a child will start breathing through her mouth. It is at this point—the change to mouth breathing during exercise—when the trouble begins in a child with exercise-induced asthma.

The nose is designed to humidify and warm inhaled air, so that the big airways in the lungs (which are sensitive to dry and cold air to a variable degree) are protected from being dried out. Breathing through the mouth *bypasses* the nose, and then the orally inhaled air is not nearly as well conditioned (humidified and warmed) when it enters the chest, especially if the breathing is heavy (as during exercise).

Dry air flowing into the airways of the chest causes the thin layer of fluid that lines the airway walls to evaporate into the air, and that dries out the airway. A couple of things happen then. First of all, it is like dry skin, and dry skin gets itchy and inflamed; the airway behaves the same way. Second, some cells that line the airway can get sick (dysfunctional) when they are dried out, and some of those cells when sick can release compounds or trigger nerve responses that cause narrowing and obstruction of the airways, including, most notably, bronchospasm and cough. It is the bronchospasm that bothers most children with

You might ask why our nose isn't better designed: biology should have sorted this out earlier by making our nose big enough to have better airflow. I think it has more to do with physics than biology. If the nose allowed airflow that was fast enough to supply the body's needs during exercise, it wouldn't be able to humidify and warm it sufficiently while at rest. And most of the time, especially in the modern world, we are at rest.

exercise-induced asthma, but coughing comes in at a close second.

Dry air and cold air share something in common: there is not much moisture in the air. So it turns out that cold air breathed through the mouth is a doubly bad insult to the airways in the chest.

It takes a few minutes for the airways in the chest to start drying out after a child has switched from nasal to oral breathing during exercise. About five minutes or so is usual. So it takes the child (with exercise-induced asthma) 5–10 minutes of exercise before the symptoms start. Those symptoms are coughing, wheezing, and shortness of breath.

If a child starts coughing and/or wheezing immediately at the onset of exercise (as opposed to it taking 5–10 minutes), it makes me think of things *other* than exercise-induced asthma. Some things I might consider include (1) insufficiently treated airflow narrowing and obstruction from other causes of asthma that is already present at the start of exercise, (2) acid reflux and aspiration (which can be worse during exercise), (3) malacia or other anatomic cause of narrowing, or (4) an entity called vocal cord syndrome. We will discuss vocal cord syndrome in the next chapter.

Some exercise gurus teach to breathe in through the nose and out through the mouth. This makes sense especially for people with exercise-induced asthma. Breathing in through the nose still is going to be difficult when oxygen demand is high in exercise, but at least breathing out (through the mouth) is more easily accomplished, and breathing *out* through the mouth is harmless.

It is not always possible to breathe in through the nose, even when you are paying attention, because the air demands get pretty high during exercise. The body does have one way to help: breathing through the nose keeps the nose decongested and more airflow can get through. Try it yourself. Next time you get a stuffy nose, try breathing through it. After you have moved ten breaths through a nostril (which can be hard to do), you probably will begin to note a substantial improvement in airflow as the engorged blood vessels in the congested nose shrink down. By the way, *not* breathing through the nose will allow the nose to congest or stay congested. If a child at rest prefers to breathe through her mouth, her nose will stay congested. Nagging a child to breathe through her nose instead of her mouth is an exercise in frustration and futility, and I don't recommend it. Instead, I recommend you ask your doctor to help identify whatever is making the nasal airflow initially poor. It could be allergies, enlarged adenoids, or an anatomic abnormality in the nose, like a deviated septum.

Exercise-induced asthma is a reasonably specific diagnosis. It can exist entirely on its own in children without any other type of asthma. Or it can occur alongside, interact with, and contribute to other types of asthma. It seems that children with allergic-inflammatory asthma are substantially more prone to exercise-induced asthma than other children are. In other words, exercise-induced asthma is more likely in kids who have asthma from other causes too.

For now, know that exercise-induced asthma causes cough and wheeze and shortness of breath that begins at least 5 minutes after the start of exercise. If that is not your child's pattern of symptoms, you should think that exercise-induced asthma is not the correct, or at least not the only, diagnosis.

Breathing slowly through the mouth at rest is not as drying to the lower airways as breathing hard and fast through the mouth is during exercise. But chronic mouth breathing is not optimal. There are many biochemical reasons to suspect that chronic mouth breathing increases asthma symptomatology. Children with untreated or improperly treated allergies may get so much nasal congestion that they *can't* breathe through their nose. (It is usually *incredibly* easy to fix nasal congestion caused by allergy, by the way.) There are other causes of chronic mouth breathing, including very enlarged adenoids, deviated nasal septum, and bony abnormalities of the nasal anatomy, that are correctable, but not so easily as allergies are to fix. Improving nasal airflow in your child with asthma (regardless of the cause of asthma) is probably going to be helpful.

CHAPTER 18

Vocal Cord Syndrome

Vocal cord syndrome is a strange entity that most commonly occurs in adult women, but can occur in older school-age children and teenagers of either sex. Statistically at least, it is not much of a problem in younger children. I really don't like the term "vocal cord syndrome," but that is one of the most common terms used to describe the condition, so I will use it here.

It is indeed a *syndrome*, meaning that it is not a disease, it doesn't have a specific cause, and it is not well understood. But vocal cord syndrome is very real, and can confuse parents and doctors alike into thinking that asthma is flaring, when it may well not be.

This condition does not primarily involve the vocal cords, but rather the larynx and the muscles that control it, and particularly the part of the larynx just above the vocal cords.

It is confused with asthma a lot, because it can show up with similar symptoms.

I know I haven't told you what vocal cord syndrome is yet. I'll get to it in a sec!

The larynx serves two primary purposes: (1) it automatically closes the airway as part of the muscular process that occurs during swallowing—this is done to prevent aspiration; (2) it supports the vocal cords for the purpose of communication. The first is most important for now: the larynx is designed for the purpose of reflexively protecting the airway from getting things down into it that will be hard to get back up, including food, fluids, saliva, and other things harmful to the airways of the chest.

If the larynx senses that something other than air is about to go down into the airway, it reflexively closes to prevent the danger of choking. That's a good larynx!

But the larynx can get confused. Occasionally a larynx is *too* protective. If the larynx is too protective, then it can reflexively close off in response to something not really dangerous to the airway, such as a strongly scented substance like perfume or the odor from a cleaning compound. When breathing in a scent, there is no liquid or food at risk of going down into the airway, but in some people, the nerves of the larynx nonetheless can get confused by the strong odor into *thinking* there is food trying to get through, and the larynx can overreact, and shut closed. When that happens, it can be very hard to breathe until the larynx opens back up again.

The symptom of this is usually the sudden (as in, *immediate*) onset of noisy difficult breathing when a strong chemical is sensed. It is not wet noise like a mucousy airway, for there is no time for the glands to secrete mucus. It is dry because it is a nerve and muscle reflex. There is no inflammation, no bronchospasm, nothing else other than the normal muscles of the larynx closing the airway for an abnormal reason.

The symptoms usually don't last long. Perhaps 20 minutes or less. But they can recur multiple times per day.

When the larynx is closed completely, no air can pass. Such complete closure *usually* lasts for only a second or two, like in a swallow. But when this *vocal cord syndrome* process is happening, the larynx stays partially closed for a lot longer, making airflow difficult. The tissue of the larynx obstructs airflow, causes it to get turbulent (noisy), and the walls vibrate, making noises that can sound a whole lot like wheezing. The vibrating tissue often can trigger coughing too .

Vocal cord syndrome can cause stridor (see sidebar), and when it does, most doctors will rapidly realize that the larynx is the culprit. However, often vocal cord syndrome sounds wheezy. And that can be confusing, especially since most doctors other than asthma specialists don't know that vocal cord syndrome even exists.

There is some degree of momentum and inertia in medicine.

Here's an example of how medical momentum can show up. A girl goes to the emergency room for sudden onset of breathing problems. (*We* know it is vocal cord syndrome because we are in the middle of a chapter on it, but the parent, child, and hospital do not know this.) The nurse at the front (triage nurse) notes that the child is oxygenating her blood just fine but the nurse hears wheezy noises and writes on the chart "wheezing." Then the nurse provides an initial medication, usually an inhaled nebulizer treatment designed to treat bronchospasm (such as albuterol), while the child waits to see the doctor. Of course, episodes of vocal cord syndrome only last minutes or maybe half an hour at a time, and so while the child is breathing the albuterol, the vocal cord syndrome settles down (just coincidentally). By the time the doctor sees the girl, she is breathing fine, the wheezy noises are gone, and everyone mistakenly attributes the improvement to the albuterol.

Now, the albuterol actually did nothing at all except take up some time while the vocal cord syndrome settled down on its own. But the child now has been witnessed to have "reversible wheezing," and there is an assumption that this came from inflamed lower airways and asthma. Remember no one measured the girl's inflammation, but doctors have been taught to assume (mistakenly) that inflammation is *always* there in a child with asthma. So the child is prescribed inhaled or oral (swallowed) anti-inflammatories (which she doesn't need) and bronchodilators (which won't help) and she leaves the emergency room with the new diagnosis of "asthma,"

> Stridor is a squeaky noise during inspiration and sometimes expiration that occurs from narrowing of the trachea or larynx. It is often homophonous but can be quite vibratory. Stridor is the noise made by a young child with croup. It is different from a wheeze. Wheeze is thinner, finer, and usually of many different pitches. Stridor is coarse, strong, and sounds like a kazoo. Wheeze from asthma is worse during expiration. Stridor is worse during inspiration. *Croup, by the way, is a term to describe inflammation and narrowing of the airway just below the vocal cords and is most commonly an issue in younger children. It is usually, but not always, caused by respiratory viruses.*

which isn't really a diagnosis and which she doesn't really have (even by my definition, because by my definition, asthma occurs in the chest, not in the larynx, which is above the chest). Next time she "wheezes" everyone will think it is "asthma" and she will probably be treated according to the asthma guidelines, which involve increasing doses and numbers of medications, none of which she actually needs and none of which will work for her. That's medical momentum.

Anyhow, vocal cord syndrome is *really* easy to misdiagnose as "asthma" and the wrong therapies are regularly provided, at higher and higher doses, until finally someone figures it out. Even subspecialist asthma doctors can occasionally get fooled by vocal cord syndrome.

Vocal cord syndrome does not involve airflow obstruction or narrowing in the chest. It does not involve airway inflammation. It does not involve allergies. It does not involve airway drying. It is an errant neurologic reflex response to a stimuli that should not, but does, cause the larynx to close.

Lots of children have asthma of various kinds, and a few children have vocal cord syndrome. Sometimes asthma and vocal cord syndrome can occur in the same child, and it can get really confusing to everybody when that is the case.

Here's what would make me likely to think about vocal cord syndrome as a problem for your child.

1. *If your child has sudden onset of wheezing that is worse with inspiration than expiration, and then it goes away over a half hour or less.*
2. *If your child is bothered by harsh smells that cause her to cough or wheeze almost immediately upon smelling them.*
3. *If your child is generally an anxious person.* Vocal cord syndrome, particularly in teenagers and adults, most commonly occurs in people who are generally anxious, and is even associated with panic attacks. By the way, the term "associated" just means that they are often seen together. This does not imply cause and effect, nor a universal association.

It is quite possible to have vocal cord syndrome without any anxiety problems at all. However, it may be worthwhile to note that when airways close off out of the blue, making it hard to breathe, such an event can provoke anxiety in a child (or an adult). It is scary to not be able to breathe. So even though anxiety is not necessarily the cause of vocal cord syndrome, anxiety can easily result from it.

4. *If there is no other evident explanation that makes sense to explain what is going on.* Vocal cord syndrome often shows up with a set of symptoms that really *don't make sense to a doctor.* Things that don't make sense deserve extra thought—indeed if things don't make sense, usually an underlying assumption is at fault. If a doctor has never heard of vocal cord syndrome, the doctor might think, "Gee, this is not quite right, but it sorta could be maybe asthma," and so it gets diagnosed as "asthma." If a doctor knows about vocal cord syndrome (knows that it exists), he is more likely to think about it.

Allergic reactions to something that is inhaled take a few minutes to start up and be noticed, because allergic reactions involve cells of the airway releasing various inflammatory compounds and that takes a bit of time to happen. Perfumes and strong scents aren't going to cause allergy in general because they aren't particularly allergenic (meaning the immune system doesn't bother with them). If you think your child seems allergic to a perfume because she coughs or wheezes when she smells it, try to note how fast the reaction happens. I bet it happens in seconds. If so, it is not allergy and much more likely to be vocal cord syndrome.

So, diagnosis of vocal cord syndrome might be made by a doctor aware of the existence of the condition and a history in a patient that seems to be consistent, when it doesn't make sense that it is anything else.

Is there diagnostic testing available that pegs the diagnosis? Sort of and sometimes. They aren't great though.

A doctor can perform laryngoscopy. Directly looking at the larynx through a laryngoscope helps a doctor make sure that the anatomy of the larynx is okay. Some doctors (I don't happen to be one of them) find that they can sometimes see abnormal closure of the larynx if they happen to view it during an episode (meaning that the patient is conscious and alert). This procedure is not comfortable or pleasant for a child, and generally does not need to be done if the only purpose is to diagnose vocal cord syndrome. It occasionally does have value, however, in ruling out other, more dangerous laryngeal abnormalities.

Spirometry can be performed. Spirometry is a form of lung-function test that I discussed in chapter 11. It is painless and pretty easy to do for children over the age of about 6 years old. Spirometry should look normal in patients with vocal cord syndrome, except if the spirometry is performed *during* an episode, when there is a specific pattern that can be seen (specifically: a limitation of *inspiratory* peak flow—which is different from the Peak *Expiratory* Flow, mentioned earlier).

Oxygen saturation testing (pulse oximetry) is particularly helpful. In vocal cord syndrome, oxygen saturations are almost always totally normal, meaning that the oxygen saturation is greater than 95 percent, even when the symptoms are very pronounced. There is a little blurb in the book on pulse oximetry in the chapter on lung-function testing.

It is uncommon for any medical test to be done during an episode of vocal cord syndrome because the episodes are short. However that doesn't have to be the case. Nowadays, you can obtain for $25 your own fingertip oxygen saturation meter. For about the same amount you can get a device that measures some of the information that spirometry measures. And maybe these inexpensive devices are worth having right in your home. They can help you help your child. But they aren't mandatory.

What do you do about treating vocal cord syndrome? Well, fortunately, it happens mostly in older children. Letting a child know what it is, that it is not dangerous, and that each episode will settle down on its own, is a great step toward curing it. Knowledge will lessen anxiety, and it is anxiety that is often the worst thing about vocal cord syndrome. Your older child may even be able to teach herself to counter the laryngeal reflex to strong scents.

During an episode you can put the oxygen-saturation monitor on.

This is not medically needed at all. Rather it is purely to help reassure you and your older child that she is oxygenating just fine. Hold her hand and tell her the episode is going to go away. Give her a nebulizer of saline (sterile salt water of a particular concentration—actually 0.9 percent— without any medicine in it) that your pharmacy can provide to you. Perhaps most importantly, have your child pretend to yawn (which helps to open the larynx). These can all lead to resolution.

If your child is an anxious person, then treating the anxiety with counseling, reassurance, proven remedies, and sometimes medications can help with vocal cord syndrome.

I think a better term for vocal cord syndrome is "intermittent hyperactive laryngeal obstruction syndrome." But I am not in charge.

The biggest danger of vocal cord syndrome is that it scares the parent and child and can get misdiagnosed by doctors. If misdiagnosed as "asthma," the doctors will see that the regular asthma medications at regular doses *do not work* for your child, and then what sometimes happens is that high-dose oral (swallowed—not inhaled) steroids are used for long periods of time to try to control the "asthma." These won't work either, but oral (swallowed) steroids have side effects, and lots of them. Long-term unnecessary use of oral steroids is perhaps the biggest danger of vocal cord syndrome, and your knowledge that vocal cord syndrome exists might save your child from those oral steroid toxicities.

As I mentioned earlier, vocal cord syndrome can be present in a child who *also* has some form of asthma. If your child seems to have both vocal cord dysfunction and asthma, it can be hard to tell what problem is causing the symptoms in any given episode. It is fine to give a bronchodilator (like albuterol) for an episode of wheezing. If it was vocal cord syndrome causing the wheezing, the dose of albuterol won't cause harm (the vocal cord syndrome will go away with time), and if it was actually asthma going on, it will probably help.

Your awareness of the existence of vocal cord syndrome, if it seems to be present in your child, will help a whole lot in getting the overall asthma and respiratory situation under control.

CHAPTER 19

Respiratory Distress

This chapter discusses signs of respiratory distress. Respiratory distress is a situation in which a child is unable to comfortably move enough air in and out of his lungs to satisfy his body's need for oxygen and to eliminate carbon dioxide. It can cause a lot of anxiety (and anxiety can actually cause respiratory distress, for that matter), in both a child and her parents.

How do you know if your child is so sick that you need to see a doctor, or go to an emergency room?

Here's the most important answer:

If you are frightened at the way your child looks, seek knowledgeable medical help. Your fright may prevent you from thinking as clearly as you should otherwise. Fright is also an indicator that you are not sure about what's up and what to do. You should seek help.

As you get more experienced with your child's asthma, you will be less frightened, and feel much more competent both in assessment and in intervention. Instead of being frightened, you will instead simply *know* when he needs to come to the emergency room or visit the doctor.

But as a parent you should take it easy on yourself, as well as be humble. You should invite the professionals in to help you whenever you aren't pretty darn sure about things. You can learn from your doctor, as well as other doctors and the nurses in clinics and emergency rooms and acute care clinics.

Respiratory distress can happen at any age, and arises from many diseases. It can occur because of asthma. I would like to present general thoughts about breathing problems in the very young (neonates and infants) before embarking on a discussion of respiratory distress in asthmatic children who are a bit older.

Breathing concerns in neonates (first month of life) and premature infants are best addressed by seeing a doctor as soon as possible. A newborn's breathing problem is *not* going to be asthma. It is far too complicated, and too dangerous, to try to teach about baby breathing problems in a book. In brief, newborn babies and small infants who are sick in *any* way (lungs or elsewhere in their body) may breathe too fast, or breathe too slow, or have long pauses of their breathing (apnea). So they can breathe too fast *or* too slow when they are sick? Yes, that's right. Additionally, newborns may have irregular, immature breathing patterns in which they change the rate of their breathing over a minute or two, up and down. That can add confusion.

It takes an experienced medical eye to figure out how sick a sick baby is. Breathing trouble in a baby can be a sign of many very different diseases that involve organs other than the lung. See your doctor if you have any concerns at all at this age. Seeing a doctor frequently in the first year of life, especially as a first-time parent (or the first time you as a parent have had a sick child), is part of parental education. Take advantage of this opportunity to learn, especially in that first month. Children are expensive, sure, but don't scrimp on getting good advice when it comes to learning about your small child's health.

Other signs that a newborn is sick also require experience to understand and figure out. Beyond strange breathing patterns or looking like he is working hard to breathe, you as a parent might notice that your baby's color is not right, or that he is grunting (a real danger sign), or his nostrils are flaring open with each breath, or that he's not eating much, or tiring rapidly when eating, or not peeing enough, or seems lethargic, dazed, or overly fussy, or smells funny. Or it could be anything that makes you concerned. Indeed, any of these occurrences *should* make you concerned.

Parental instincts have been honed over the history of humanity's existence on the planet, so the default answer is to trust your instincts if they are telling you to be worried. If you are worried, seek help.

After the neonatal period (after one month of age), infants start getting more resilient. And so do parents. You will know your baby better and you will be better able to recognize normal from abnormal more confidently. All this is good. Still, err on the side of seeking advice.

Infants will reveal narrowed or sick airways or lungs with wheezing and coughing. However, they may also display the following signs of respiratory distress:

- Poor feeding
- Lethargy (or persistent fussiness)
- Rapid breathing
- Hard work of breathing (abdomen and chest see-sawing, retractions between ribs during inhalation)
- Grunting (the infant will pause after inhalation and then blow out her first bit of exhalation with a grunting sound. Danger!)
- Nasal flaring (the nostrils open wider with each breath)
- Skin color not pink (perhaps even gray or with a bluish tone—danger!)

All these are reasons to seek help right away for your baby.

Preschool children will show some of the same signs as infants, but children this age can communicate a bit better, and you will fully know your child's cues by this age. Wheeze and cough and fussiness and loss of activity and rapid breathing are potential signs of asthma acting up. Children sick with asthma won't run around for as long as usual before they tire out. They will get short of breath, or have to cough a lot when they run.

School-age children with asthma out of control will cough and wheeze, often with a wet mucousy chest. Coughing at night is a common early sign of asthma flaring. As the asthma exacerbation progresses, a child will tire easily, and can't run for long. As the asthma further worsens, a child cannot climb a flight of stairs without having to recover for quite a while afterward. This inability to climb stairs without getting tired out is a solid sign of troublesome airflow limitation, or something else that also needs medical attention.

Wheezing is a sign of obstruction and narrowing. And when it is bad, it can be evidence of respiratory distress. The *cessation* of wheezing in a child who is still having trouble breathing is a worrisome sign. When children stop wheezing but still look bad, it does *not* mean they are getting better. Instead, it may likely mean that the airways obstructions are getting *complete* and air is flowing too little even to make wheezing noises. This is trouble.

Respiratory distress is a scary thing, and rightfully so. If you are scared, or your child is scared, seek help.

Again, you'll get better and better at figuring things out over time. Take the opportunities to learn from experts.

CHAPTER 20

What about "Bronchitis" and "Sinusitis"?

Everyone has heard of bronchitis. But what is it? Remember, "-itis" at the end of an anatomic term means *inflammation*. Bronch*itis* is therefore just *inflammation of the bronchi*. Indeed *asthma from allergic inflammation from sensitivity to dust mites* is a form of bronchitis. *Viral-induced asthma* is a form of bronchitis too. Even though many people think that bronchitis is something you treat with antibiotics, neither of these most common causes of asthma should be treated with antibiotics.

Antibiotics treat bacterial infections, not the common cold, and not allergies.

We have all heard that antibiotic overuse (for inappropriate treatment of viruses and for helping food animals like cows and chickens grow better) leads to resistance forming to the antibiotics. Resistance to antibiotics is a trait of bacteria, not humans. If a certain antibiotic has not helped your child in the past, that does not mean that *your child* is resistant to the good effects of an antibiotic. Rather it means something else. It may mean that the cause of the illness (for which the antibiotic did not work in your child) was actually a virus or something nonbacterial, like the common cold, for which

Asthmatic bronchitis is a term that is occasionally used for "asthma" and in my mind would be a great term for *inflammatory* types of asthma. Yet I don't tend to use this term. The term can lead to confusion because most patients and parents errantly think that *bronchitis* is supposed to be treated with antibiotics, even though bronchitis just means inflammation from any cause (bacterial or otherwise).

131

Sinuses are not the same thing as the *nose*. Sinuses are air spaces within the skull bones that connect by little tubes into the nasal airway. There are sinuses under the cheek-bones (maxillary sinus), above the eyes (frontal sinus) and deep back behind the nose (ethmoid and sphenoid sinuses). The sinuses lighten the weight of the skull and change the tone of speech. If the tube connecting a sinus to the nose gets obstructed, sinus inflammation and infection with bacteria can result.

of course the antibiotic could not possibly work. Or it might mean that the bacteria that made your child sick that time was resistant to that antibiotic. There is a lot of debate and thought about antibiotic use in children, and it is more than this book can deal with.

But it is fair in this book to ask you not to pressure your doctor for antibiotics when your doctor is confident that a virus or allergies are causing your child's troubles. Doctors will cave under pressure: they want to keep you happy. But it would be better if you would be happy with your doctor because he *protected* you from wasting money on antibiotics, or protected your child from risking side effects from them.

In fact, in children, bronchitis seems to be only rarely bacterial. Bronchial inflammation (bronchitis) is usually viral in otherwise healthy children, or allergic in children with allergic inflammatory asthma. Bacterial bronchitis can occur in children, but when it happens more than once or twice in otherwise seemingly healthy children, I do raise my eyebrows. Recurrent bacterial bronchitis in children makes me wonder about underlying abnormalities in their airways, such as cystic fibrosis or immune deficiencies or tobacco-smoke exposure or anatomic abnormalities, or other problems that prevent inhaled or aspirated bacteria from being cleared out by the normal mechanisms that protect airways from inhaled yuk.

Our ability to know for sure whether respiratory infections are bacterial or viral is *very limited indeed*. Actually, physicians are usually, or even almost always, guessing. Is this a cold in the nose, or a bacterial sinusitis causing all the boogers and the fussiness? Is this a virus in the bronchi or a bacterial infection or allergic inflammation causing all that coughing and wheezing? We often *just don't know*.

In this regard, each doctor uses a decision-making system that he has found works for him. I developed my system too. It is only a guide, though, and I alter it depending on the child or circumstances.

For example, in regard to sinus problems, if a child has fever and runny nose, it is likely (nine times out of ten) going to be a cold virus that is responsible. If the cold symptoms are not improving by 10–14 days like they should, it may be either a second cold has been picked up, or indeed it might be a bacterial sinusitis, so I might prescribe antibiotics after two weeks of persistent unimproving cold symptoms. Yes, had we treated with antibiotics sooner, the child might have been better faster. But if we treated all kids with cold symptoms with antibiotics, just in case it might be a bacterial sinusitis, we would have even more bacterial resistance on our hands, and lots of children would have unnecessarily experienced side effects of the antibiotics (including, even, allergy to them).

I also have a system for bronchitis and bronchiolitis. A first episode of bronchiolitis is almost always (but not always) caused by a virus. As is the second and third episode. A child who has 2–3 or more episodes of bronchitis or bronchiolitis has "recurrent episodes of reversible airflow limitation," or "asthma," and I will want to try to figure out what is causing it. It could be viral-induced asthma, or allergic-inflammatory asthma, or reflux asthma. Or it could be bacterial bronchitis causing the asthma.

Children with normal airways and airway function do not get recurrent bacterial infections in the airway, so I seek a possible diagnosis as to why a child might have such bacterial infections. The most common and concerning causes of recurrent *bacterial* bronchitis in children

Bacterial sinusitis (inflammation of the sinuses caused by bacteria) seems to make asthma worse in many children. Sometimes, a doctor might treat a child for "presumed sinusitis" with antibiotics to see if it helps the asthma. These are mildly tough decisions to make for a doctor because there are just no good ways to diagnose bacterial sinusitis accurately without uncomfortable tests done by an ear/nose/throat surgeon (otolaryngologist). Sometimes, doctors just have to guess. And that is okay too, as long as they are guessing what is best for *your child* when they are making their guesses.

There appears to be a subset of patients whose asthma is *caused* or *exacerbated* by certain types of bacteria that conceivably chronically infect otherwise-healthy lungs and are hard to test for. These infections are not acute and do not cause fevers. We as yet know little about the role these bacteria play in asthma. Your child's doctor may prescribe antibiotics as a trial if she thinks it is a reasonable possibility that these bacteria are relevant to your child. But your doctor is not likely to try antibiotics for this more than once or twice.

are very briefly discussed in the next chapter and include:

• Cystic fibrosis
• Antibody deficiency (immune deficiency)
• Anatomic abnormality of the airway or lung
• Dysfunction of the airway cilia (those hair cells that sweep along to propel mucus and captured particles out of the lung)

In an otherwise healthy-looking child, I might let a child "get away" with having suspected bacterial bronchitis once. But I will be thinking hard and plan to go hunting for a diagnosis as to why your child might have *recurrent* bacterial bronchitis, including evaluating for these disorders mentioned above.

Take -home message: if your child has recurrent bronchitis, it is probably not bacterial. But it could be. If it is thought to be bacterial, you need to know why it is happening. Thus, if your child is prescribed antibiotics for repeated episodes of bacterial bronchitis, you should ask your doctor to help you diagnose the cause in your child. It will be important to know. Usually such a diagnostic process means a referral to a pediatric lung specialist or an allergist/immunologist.

CHAPTER 21

Confounding Diagnoses

Asthma is not a diagnosis, but a physiologic disturbance caused by all sorts of things.

The most common entities that lead to asthma in children include:

- Viral-induced asthma (in younger children)
- Asthma from allergic airway inflammation (this increases in likelihood as children get older)
- Exercise-induced asthma (this can stand alone, or occur with virus-induced asthma or with allergic airway inflammation)

There are lots of entities that can confound or add to the symptoms of asthma in children. Some are minor, and some are more concerning. Some of these entities cause airway obstruction that lead to symptoms similar to the above three most common causes of asthma. Yet they are very different diseases, and need totally different therapies. Because the symptoms are so similar, these entities are often confused or missed, or diagnoses delayed in children who have asthma symptoms.

Stomach acid reflux can add to the asthma from other causes, or be a stand-alone cause of asthma. Malacia (floppy airways) can be present with asthma, or without asthma. Vocal cord syndrome can be readily confused with asthma, as can foreign bodies that get inhaled into the airway.

There are also troublesome chronic diseases that can cause asthma-like symptoms and you'll want to know if they are present. In fact, I mentioned them already. These troublesome diseases tend to cause recurrent episodes of bacterial bronchitis.

These entities include cystic fibrosis (CF) — a genetic condition that leads to dysfunction of the gut that prevents normal absorption of food, and dysfunction of the airways that leads to lung disease with airflow limitation. Cystic fibrosis is often identified in newborn screening tests performed in the first days of life. Children with untreated CF tend to be skinny, usually have lots of loose stool every day, and develop chronic respiratory symptoms including coughing and mucus production. There are about 40,000 people in the US with CF. It is sometimes initially confused with causes of asthma, but CF needs entirely different treatment. Your doctor should at least consider the possibility of CF in any child with asthma. Most doctors will quickly run it through their mind (as they do with many possible diagnoses) and likely will not mention CF at all if he thinks it is unlikely in your child. Certainly you can and should ask your doctor if he thinks CF is possible. I won't get further into CF in this book.

Immune deficiencies, including low or absent levels of certain antibodies, can lead to lung disease with airflow limitation that can be confused with various causes of asthma. These immune deficiencies allow for bacterial infections to occur in the lungs. Bacterial infections are not commonly involved in allergic or viral-induced asthma but *are* important contributors to lung disease that results from immune deficiency.

Antibody deficiencies can allow bacterial bronchitis to occur (which causes asthma symptoms but is not treated the way other causes of asthma are) as well as pneumonia and repeated bouts with sinusitis and ear infections. You should ask your doctor about the possibility of immune deficiencies if your child has recurrent ear infections, sinusitis, and bacterial bronchitis and pneumonia. That immune deficiencies exist in the world and may cause asthma symptoms does not mean that any formal testing must be used to seek them in *your* child. Sometimes it is appropriate to look (with blood tests) and sometimes it is fine to wait and see, and test later if needed. Your doctor or a specialist will know.

Certainly it is more common for a child to have allergic asthma causing bronchitis and to have allergies causing sinusitis than it is to have immune deficiencies. It is also still common to have these allergic causes misdiagnosed as bacterial.

Dysfunction of the cilia cells (hair cells) in the lungs can happen because of a genetic disease (*primary ciliary dyskinesia*), or because of other problems. It is sometimes called *immotile cilia syndrome*, which is a broader term we use when we don't yet know whether it is genetic or the result of other diseases of the airway. When the cilia don't function correctly, mucus is not cleared well from the lungs, nor from the sinuses and middle ear spaces. Recurrent bacterial infections of the airways, lungs, sinuses, and ears result (very similar to how antibody deficiencies show up!). Testing for ciliary dyskinesia can be done with a simple quick brushing sample taken from the nose right in the office in seconds, without any need for sedation. But because of the nature of the way the sample is then examined in the lab, this test is usually only done by specialists (pediatric pulmonologists, otolaryngologists, and some allergists) at university hospitals who have access to the laboratory pathologists who know what to look for. It's actually an easy test, but most doctors have never seen it done!

There can be tumors inside the airways or outside the airways. They are not common. Often the tumors are not cancerous, but that doesn't mean they don't cause trouble. They can be initially confused with the causes of asthma, because these tumors can cause wheezing and coughing or other respiratory noises. They don't go away with the usual treatments used in children with asthma, but one or two of them can get better temporarily with oral (swallowed) steroids, so they can be confusing to diagnose.

My rule of thumb is that a first-time wheezing child deserves an x-ray to make sure her anatomy is okay and there are no tumors. My other rule of thumb is that if a child is not getting better with optimum treatment for the diagnoses that I made, or not following an expected pattern for the disease I diagnosed, then I have to rethink the diagnosis, for it might have been wrong. For example, if I treat a child for allergic inflammation and his asthma gets no better, I need to look for other diagnoses.

Obesity is a risk factor for asthma. Obesity does not seem to be a particularly big risk factor for *allergy*, nor therefore for allergic inflammatory asthma. (By the way, that means that obesity doesn't *increase* the risk of allergy or allergic inflammatory asthma, but an obese child can still have allergy).

If your school-age child is obese, and has asthma, of course check for allergies, and if present, seek to control allergic inflammation. But if asthma symptoms still persist, consider other things. Stomach acid reflux is worse in children who are obese, and may contribute to asthma. The airways may be a bit narrower in obesity and the demand for airflow during exercise higher, which makes *relative* narrowing and resulting wheezing more likely. Also, certain markers of inflammation are found to be higher in many obese people, so it may be that obese children might have more pronounced non-allergic inflammation in their airways. Asthma associated with obesity is often harder to manage than allergic inflammatory asthma, in part because we often don't understand it.

CHAPTER 22

Allergic Bronchopulmonary Aspergillosis (ABPA)

What's that you say? ABPA? What on earth is that, and I don't want it! Aspergillus is a mold that is all over the place: indoors some, outdoors lots. You can't get rid of it without nuking the whole planet surface, and I would ask you not to do that.

It is reasonably common to be allergic to aspergillus. In some allergic children (not many, fortunately) a combination of uncertain factors leads them (1) to be allergic to aspergillus, (2) to get a little aspergillus inhaled into the lungs, and (3) to respond to this aspergillus with lots of allergic airway inflammation, mucus production, and airway obstruction, which then in turn allows for (4) the growth of more aspergillus right within the lung itself. Bronchopulmonary means "bronchial airways and the lungs," and this is where the ABPA process occurs.

Now, aspergillus doesn't cause disease in most healthy people. We can and do inhale it and our cilia clear it. But in a person who has something abnormal about her airway (such as cystic fibrosis) and develops allergy to aspergillus, there is trouble. ABPA can also happen in children with allergic inflammatory asthma, which in some children can interfere with airway function sufficiently to allow aspergillus to start its evil assault.

ABPA is very common in children with cystic fibrosis (most children with CF have allergies). ABPA is less common in children with the more typical causes of asthma. It is quite rare in an asthmatic child under age 7 years (but can happen).

139

Now is a good time to wax philosophical about medical specialists. I'm a specialist, so I can make light of myself. Specialists know a huge amount about very little. Generalist doctors (like family-practice docs and pediatricians) know a good bit about a whole ton of things. The generalists refer patients to the specialists when they need their expertise, but few specialists are able to help with all the medical needs of a child. A generalist should usually be your child's principal doctor. But ABPA requires a specialist.

Imagine being allergic to a cat, and having a cat living in your lungs. That would be bad. ABPA is rather like that, except that it is a mold in the lungs.

When might you suspect your school-age child has ABPA? Well, if for years your child's asthma has been pretty well controlled and not much of a problem, and then over a period of months the asthma gets way out of control and he starts having repeated bad asthma episodes that require long courses of oral steroids, you need to suspect ABPA.

Now, there are a lot of doctors out there who do not know about ABPA because it is not that common. So you may need to mention it to your doctor (you and your child's doctor work in a partnership, remember). In my opinion ABPA needs to be evaluated, diagnosed, and managed by an allergist or a pediatric pulmonologist. Testing for it requires skin and blood allergy tests, sputum analysis if possible, a CT scan of the chest, lung-function testing, and specialist-level experience to sort it all out.

Treatment of ABPA is with long-term therapy against allergic inflammation, combined often with a medication that kills the mold. This therapy is beyond the scope of this book, for sure, but often involves many, many months of oral (swallowed) steroids, and all the side effects that come with those. You need an allergist or a pediatric pulmonologist to manage this. Either specialist will be able to guide the therapy.

Fortunately it is very unlikely your child will ever have ABPA! I just want you to know about it in case your older child, out of the blue, starts getting much worse episodes of asthma than he used to have, over and over again.

CHAPTER 23

Putting the Diagnostic Pieces Together

The diagnoses that underlie asthma symptoms that we have discussed so far include

1. Viral-induced asthma (usually in infants and preschoolers)
2. Allergic inflammatory asthma caused by inhaled allergens (commonly also with viral triggering of episodes)
3. Exercise-induced asthma
4. Irritant-induced asthma (chlorine, cigarette smoke)
5. Other causes of asthma symptoms:
    a. Narrow airways
    b. Airway malacia
    c. Stomach acid reflux

And I have mentioned some of the possible diagnoses that can get confused with asthma:

• Foreign bodies in the airway
• Tumors
• Airway anatomic defects including fistula and mislocated large arteries
• Cystic fibrosis
• Immotile cilia syndrome
• Immune deficiencies (usually antibody deficiencies)
• Allergic bronchopulmonary aspergillosis

How do we sort among them?

The answer is: a bit imperfectly. The diagnoses are accomplished with a combination of your child's doctor's knowledge of asthma and your knowledge of your child. And now also, your knowledge of asthma is added to the list of assets.

One of our best diagnostic allies is *time*. Time teaches us a lot. Time passes during a diagnostic empiric trial of medicine and we learn how a child responds to it. Time helps us see how well a child grows, how well he tolerates his respiratory problems.

In making the diagnosis of what is causing your child's asthma, the first thing I would suggest is that you ask yourself what types of asthma that you have read about so far in this book seem to most accurately describe what you see in your child. Also ask yourself what things I have mentioned that *look* like asthma, or are confused with asthma, that you found yourself wondering about.

Then let's think through asthma based on your child's age.

Starting in *infancy*.

If your child has asthma symptoms (RAD?) as an infant, and gets sick in his chest when he gets colds, then probably your child has viral-induced asthma, or possibly malacia, or also possibly congenitally small or narrowed airways.

If your small child makes all sorts of noises in the airway when he doesn't have a cold, when he is excited and enthusiastic for example, then he may well have malacia. Malacia noises can come and go quickly depending on how your child is breathing, but can persist when there is a cold. Children with malacia are often "happy wheezers," with intermittent symptoms occurring here and there and not lasting long (maybe ten minutes at a time). This contrasts with viral-infection wheezing, which tends to persist for days.

Congenitally narrow airways are not diagnosable directly unless there is something highly abnormal about a child's airway cartilage. It is something we guess might be the case in a small child who, when healthy, breathes faster than other infants and works a bit harder to breathe than others when he gets excited or mad, but who doesn't have the coarse kazooey floppy airway noises of malacia.

And how about stomach acid reflux? Most babies reflux. If your infant is a wet-burpy baby (which confirms reflux without any tests whatsoever!) and he has lots of wheezing, then reflux might well be a factor in his asthma. But to know for sure? Well, not much is for sure, but you can come close. You can try a diagnostic empiric trial.

For the *acid* component of reflux (which is most often the major player because it triggers all that inflammation stuff), your doctor may prescribe a couple of weeks of stomach-acid-blocking medicine and see how it works. When I start such an empiric trial, I prefer to use a pretty strong dose of a class of drug called proton pump inhibitors. These drugs—including Prilosec (omeprazole), Nexium (esomeprazole), Prevacid (lansoprazole), and others—work by blocking the acid pumps in the stomach that get turned on after a meal. These drugs work best by far if they are given 45 minutes *before* a meal.

For this empiric trial, we want to suppress stomach acid as much as possible, because we are testing to see if acid is relevant. So suppress it with a good solid dose of the medication(s). Then, in a week or two, watch to see if there is a huge improvement in the chronic respiratory symptoms. If there is, then probably (or at least maybe) the stomach acid is playing a role. (It could also be that your child was going to be getting better anyway just then, so it *is* possible to be faked out by an empiric trial. But it is better by far than just guessing.) Then, if it seems pretty likely that the diagnostic empiric trial worked, your child can have a diagnosis of "likely acid reflux–induced asthma." With a reasonable diagnosis in hand, it is fine to lower the dose of acid blocking medicine to the lowest dose that stays effective.

It is also possible that the acid-blockade medicine causes no improvement in your child at all. If that is the case, it is unlikely that he has acid reflux–induced asthma (at this time at least). His symptoms still could come from aspiration of milk or food though (as opposed to acid). This can be assessed with a radiographic procedure called a "milk scan" done in a special part of radiology (x-ray) facilities, or with the help of a pediatric pulmonologist. And there are some things that your doctor can advise you to do to help lessen reflux in infants, such as thickening of feeds, burping more frequently and changing feeding position.

Allergy testing can be done in your infant, but it is rarely (almost never) useful to check for inhalant allergies. Instead, the focus is on some common foods, such as milk, egg, soy, and a few other things. Conceivably, your child could have allergic airway inflammation from reflux and aspiration of foods he eats and is allergic to.

By the way, if your child has eczema and is allergic to milk or egg or soy or some other food, then he will probably develop allergies to inhaled stuff later (within a few years), so you will want to do more allergy testing over the years.

Your doctor can help you think through the *confounders of asthma*— the other diseases like antibody deficiencies, cystic fibrosis, and immotile cilia syndrome that show up in infancy and can be confused with the common causes of asthma.

Children who have respiratory disease and do not gain weight well are a particular concern. Such children may have a disease that needs the help of a pediatric lung specialist to diagnose and manage. Often these other diagnoses are more of a challenge to a child than the common causes of asthma are, and so the child struggles more with them. Breathing troubles in the setting of poor weight gain is a reason to seek subspecialist advice.

Let's move on to the *preschool-age children*.

These children are usually outgrowing malacia if they had it, and their airways are bigger now so that small airways are less of an issue. At this age, viral-induced asthma dominates statistically, reflux plays a role in some children, and asthma from allergic airway inflammation caused by inhalant allergies starts to appear.

By the time your child is perhaps 2-3 years old, it is reasonable to consider testing for inhalant allergies. Allergy testing is helpful to predict the future. For example, the older *non-allergic* child with asthma usually has the same causes of asthma he had as an infant, and those types of asthma gradually get better as the years pass, and usually go away altogether.

Keep in mind that you may need to do further allergy testing as your child gets older. Usually by age 6 years, if allergies are not evident on allergy testing, your child's asthma won't be allergic in nature at all.

If your child is proven to have allergies to inhaled stuff, then it is very likely that one of the causes of her asthma is *allergic airway inflammation* and the consequences that result from it (including swelling, bronchial hyperreactivity, bronchospasm, glandular secretion, and injury to the airway wall). As children move from 2 years to 6 years, *viral-induced asthma* becomes less common, and *allergic inflammatory asthma* takes the fore (in allergic children).

I do want to reiterate that *viral-induced asthma* is different from the similar-sounding term *viral-triggering of asthma*. As you know, *allergic inflammatory asthma* is a different disease than *viral-induced asthma*. But the main trigger for an asthma exacerbation in children with *allergic inflammatory asthma* is still the common cold. This is called *viral-triggering of allergic inflammatory asthma*.

One of the differences between *viral-induced asthma* and *viral-triggering of allergic inflammatory asthma* is that the allergic inflammatory asthma is readily treated with inhaled steroid medications, and the inhaled steroids work to make children better even in the setting of viral triggering. This contrasts with *viral-induced asthma*, in which allergic inflammation is not involved, and for which steroids are usually not effective.

There is often overlap between the different causes of asthma during the late preschool and early school-age years.

As children get further into their *school-age* years, *viral-induced asthma* disappears and the children with ongoing asthma problems mostly have *allergic inflammatory asthma* (usually with viral-triggering). If your child has ongoing asthma problems at age 7 to 9 years and is *not* allergic, then it is wise to look for other causes of asthma, including anatomic abnormalities of the airway, stomach reflux, foreign bodies that may have been in the airways for months or years, irritation from smoke, and other confounders. There may well be no other causes, and it all may still be viral-induced asthma that has stuck around since infancy. But it is time to go looking.

CHAPTER 24

Introduction to Treatment

It's time finally to move on to treatment.

It now goes without saying (but I will say it anyway) that I am not a supporter of any one-size-fits-all therapeutic regimen or plan for the management of asthma in children. I hope that what you want is a treatment plan designed for *your* child, created by you and your child's doctor, both of whom know your child and care for your child. This sort of individualization of care for your child is precisely what makes sense to want, so want it! This applies both in the setting of chronic treatment of asthma (prevention and maintenance therapy) and for therapy for acute exacerbations of asthma.

The therapy this book focuses on is the chronic management of asthma and prevention of asthma flares. There are also tricks that I will recommend for dealing with acute exacerbations of asthma.

There are several items to consider when deciding on therapeutic plans for the chronic treatment of asthma:

1. The diagnosis, or several diagnoses, that cause your child's asthma
2. How much trouble your child has with asthma
3. The age of your child and ability to participate in the plan
4. The realistic possibilities to alter environment to limit allergen and irritant exposure when relevant
5. The cost of the various therapies or interventions
6. The time it takes to accomplish them

The first step is to establish the diagnosis or diagnoses underlying your child's asthma. So far, this book has been mostly about diagnosis, because getting the diagnosis correct is so important in picking out therapies and interventions. All the background offered in this book will help you assist your child's doctor in figuring out the diagnosis. You wouldn't want to treat diarrhea as if it were caused by a virus (no medication needed), when it was really caused by an intestinal parasite infection that needs to be treated with medicine. Just so for asthma.

The diagnosis/diagnoses in your child may not necessarily be apparent right away. It often takes time to get it right, and the causes of the asthma in your child can change over time. Asthma changes over time. Time is one of our best diagnostic allies. When we use a diagnostic empiric trial, it takes some time (days to weeks usually) to assess the results of a medication or an intervention. That being said, it is great to try to get it right as fast as possible. Just don't expect perfection.

There is no perfection in medicine. In medicine, what you should seek is sincere caring, professional knowledge, wise decision-making, a willingness to listen, thoughtfulness, and the ability to "think outside the box." Right now the most troublesome restricting box in society is that we are taught to think about groups, not about individuals. So it is important to get out of that box as quickly as we can.

One box is that our medical system often focuses on prescribing medication, as opposed to altering lifestyle or exposures. Swallowing pills is easier than altering lifestyle. Medications can be *absolutely wonderful* in helping your child deal with her asthma, and I will encourage their use, where appropriate, with great vigor. But medications aren't the only, or necessarily most important, intervention.

Therefore, the first part of therapy that I would like to introduce is environmental control.

CHAPTER 25

Control of the Environment

Environmental control can be extremely helpful for the management of asthma and prevention of exacerbations, but its success depends on the diagnosis or diagnoses of what is causing your child's asthma. The first part of this chapter will be focused on allergies (which are more relevant over age 3 years). The second part will discuss other environmental insults to the airways that are relevant in younger and older children alike.

I have a general rule that is almost always acceptable to follow. It is this: don't change your life in *major* ways in order to avoid allergy exposure, unless the allergic inflammation is bad and not controlled with all the various therapies we have available. Changing things in *minor* ways may be helpful however and is often wise.

If your child has allergic inflammatory asthma, then your child will have had allergy testing performed in order to establish that diagnosis correctly. You have a good idea what he is allergic to and what is causing the asthma problems.

There are indoor allergens and outdoor allergens.

For outdoor allergens, you cannot limit exposure without locking your child in a bubble or moving to Antarctica.

However, if your child is allergic to leaf mold and has lots of asthma problems in the fall, I recommend not allowing him to jump in piles of rotting leaves. Jumping in leaf piles is a ball, however, so don't stop him without thinking about it some.

Certainly some geographic locations have fewer outdoor allergens—usually dry climates are best—but a home move solely for the reasons of avoiding allergens is usually not merited.

In contrast to *outdoor* allergens, we *can* reduce levels of *indoor* allergens. If your child is allergic to indoor allergens (dust mite, cat, dog, cockroach, some molds) then there is likely some value in controlling the allergens to which he is allergic.

Dust Mites

If your child is allergic to dust mites (a very common allergy indeed), then I recommend getting *dust-mite-impermeable* pillow covers and a mattress cover for his bed. These help keep dust mites *inside* the pillow and mattress, instead of directly near your child's face. These covers prevent your child from being face first in dust mite allergen (which is, yup, dust mite poop). The pillow cover will cost between $5 and $20, and the mattress cover between $18 and $80. This is probably the single most important environmental-control effort you can do.

Then, start washing the sheets in *hot* water each week. Use *hot* water (120 degrees) because heat kills dust mites. Keep the bedclothes to a minimum, and made of material that tolerates washing in hot water too. Wash them every couple of weeks. Stuffed animals in bed should be washable in hot water and dryable in a hot dryer, or alternatively, they should be *freezable* (freezing kills dust mites too). To freeze, place the stuffed animal in a sealed plastic bag (like a big Ziploc bag) and stick it in your freezer for half a day. Then remove it from the freezer and let it warm up entirely while *still sealed in the plastic bag* so that condensation doesn't get on the toy. Dust mites love moisture and hate excessive heat and cold. They thrive in the fall more than any other season, but are considered perennial (year-round) allergens.

Oh, by the way, *hot* water also scalds children who turn on the hot faucet. Most pediatricians recommend keeping your hot water heater below 120 degrees to avoid accidental burns. But dust mites die *above* 120 degrees and your washing machine won't get hot enough if your water heater is set lower. All I can say about this is "be careful, be wise, be aware."

There are all sorts of products sold for controlling dust mites. I am open to anything, but only if it is needed. Don't be guilted into spending oodles of your hard-earned money. I would suggest that you never *increase* the amount of wall-to-wall carpeting in your home. Carpets are big dust collectors, and wall-to-wall carpets are difficult to clean effectively. In fact, steaming carpets probably doesn't heat up the dust mites enough to kill them, but gives them lots of nice moisture to breed in, so steaming isn't usually warranted. If you can cheaply get rid of carpets (wall to wall or other) in your child's room, I think it is reasonable to do so.

How about Cats?

If your child is allergic to cats, and you don't already have a cat, then don't get a cat. If your child is allergic to cats, don't even *think* about getting a cat. Cat allergen is particularly troublesome for asthma in children who are allergic to cat. Don't let a cat in the house at all. Cat dander even from a brief cat visit (like the cat of a visiting family member), will cling to the walls and ceiling and pop off to float around a room even months after the cat is gone. Outdoor cats that always stay outdoors and *never* come inside (even in a hurricane, tornado, cyclone) are fine.

What if you already have an indoor cat? Well, what can I say? Don't get another cat. I understand that cats are members of the family. You can't kick your husband or wife or children out of the house any more than you can kick your family cat out.

But what can you do to protect your child's airways from the adverse effects of your indoor cat? A few things:

1. *Never* let the cat in your child's bedroom.
2. Put a HEPA filtration device or other airborne-allergen-trapping device in your child's bedroom and run it.
3. Shave your cat naked and laugh at it. *(Okay, skip this step.)*
4. Some say wash your cat regularly. I don't know what regularly even means, and I don't know how to wash a cat. I do know that washing cats to control dander has been studied and it didn't do enough good to be worth the effort.
5. There are some supposedly hypoallergenic cats now. "Technology" is progressing. I suppose it is fine to look into them, skeptically.

Lastly, if you don't have a cat and your child is *not* allergic to cats, but *is* allergic to other things, I still recommend not getting a cat. Allergies develop over time in children and if your allergic child is not allergic to cats yet, he may still develop cat allergy later.

What about Dogs?

Dogs are not as straightforward as cats. Every child is different, and dogs are different too. Generally (but not always), dog allergy is not as bad as cat allergy, and there are clearly some species that seem truly less allergenic (which means mostly that they spread less dander around). Older dogs shed more dander than younger ones, and dogs with fur shed more than dogs with hair (but every dog is different!).

Anyhow, if your child isn't allergic to dogs, don't worry about it. It is, in my opinion, okay to get a dog. Dogs are awesome. If your child is allergic to other things, it is probably wise to get a hypoallergenic dog with hair as opposed to fur, because it is still possible your child will develop an allergy to dogs later. I recommend you do some research.

Cockroaches?

I love animals. I have empathy even to ants. I hate mosquitoes. And cockroaches? Cockroaches need to die. Cockroaches create a wicked little allergen. But they are controllable, with effort, most of the time, in most places. Yes, I know you can't always win when the neighbor in the next apartment is a bum who leaves food all over the place and his cockroaches come over to your place from time to time. But try to control your *own* cockroach risks. Don't leave food out. Empty the trash. Clean the place. And kill the cockroaches with pesticides (green or otherwise), until they are dead, dead, dead.

How about Molds?

Molds are a source of great confusion and conflicting information. Lots of allergic children are *not* allergic to molds. Mold allergy gets more common in adulthood. But some children have mold allergy, and if your child happens to be one who does, you should be aware and do what you can about mold. I recommend that you don't go overboard here. You should be skeptical about hype regarding mold. Those who clean mold for a living assuredly will tell you how dangerous mold is. But they have a conflict of interest. Really, mold is only rarely "dangerous."

Mold is everywhere. It is. Inside and outside. Invisible and visible. You can pay thousands of dollars to a company selling mold-remediation services, and they will probably clear out some percentage of the mold, but it will also probably be back within a few months. Or sooner.

You should clean up obvious, visible mold. It's nasty. In the bathrooms is a usual visible location. Around windows in your child's room too. Mold likes moisture. Lysol spray is pretty good at killing mold. There are probably fifty times more sources of invisible mold than visible mold, and you can't deal with it all, especially in your ducts, your air conditioning, and behind your walls. The professionals can help with this, but again, the cost-reward ratio is only sometimes going to be worth it.

Certainly look into the various options for cleaning mold. But know that you can never entirely eliminate molds, no matter how much money you spend! I recommend saving your money unless your doctor insists otherwise. (Remember, most likely, I haven't met you or your child, and you and your doctor need to consider *your* unique situation). I wouldn't risk ozone generators for mold remediation. Ozone is good at eliminating smells, but not good at killing molds. And ozone can cause harm to pets, houseplants, and anyone who is around.

A last note on mold. Indoor mold can cause illnesses other than allergies. When it causes other types of illness, mold remediation may well be necessary. Certain specific molds release volatile chemicals that cause harm. It is not allergy, but these can cause respiratory difficulties (and very occasionally, these can be confused with other causes of asthma). It may be possible to eradicate those molds with either inexpensive means, or expensive professional remediation. Again, that is a rare case. Whenever there is hype about anything, the truth becomes very hard to discover. There is lots of hype about molds in buildings, schools, and homes, and the truth is therefore pretty opaque.

Mice and Rats?

It is unlikely your child will be tested for allergies to rats and mice and other little critters unless you tell the doctor you have them in your house. Furry *non*-pets should be eliminated. Get a cat! (Actually, don't get a cat.) Little furry *pets* to which your child is allergic should be dealt with as you see fit, keeping them out of your child's room at the very least, and when nature calls one of these critters to its maker, it is best not to replace it with another.

In summary, control indoor allergens when you reasonably can, using the most effective and least expensive methods first. If your child is allergic to dust mites, 80% of the battle is won with a dust mite-proof pillow cover and mattress cover and by keeping the bedclothes washed. Pulling up the carpets and leaving a wood floor, if possible, is a great next step. Chemicals and expensive devices are rarely useful. Cats are trouble for children who are allergic to them or will become allergic to them. Don't underestimate the trouble caused by a cat in a child with asthma who is allergic to cat. I recommend not being in denial, nor making excuses about the cat. Deal with the issue head on with rationality and care. HEPA or other good air filtration is helpful when a cat is in the house.

If your child is chronically sick with uncontrollable allergic inflammatory asthma and is allergic to cats, and you have a cat in the house, you almost assuredly need to do something about that cat. And I am very sorry about that. My sister loves cats. She's allergic to them. And she denies it adamantly, so I understand. I am allergic to cats. Our cat made me sick for a decade, even as a young doctor. Best thing that ever happened to me, in terms of my asthma, was moving overseas where the cat was not allowed to go. I got lung healthy for the first time ever.

Non-Allergy-Related Environmental Issues That Are Potentially Relevant to Your Child's Asthma

Whether or not your child's asthma is caused by allergic inflammation, there are environmental exposures that might (*might*) be causing or worsening the asthmatic airflow limitation (in other words, might be making your child sicker).

These things are not easy to test for in a clinic nor prove with assured confidence in an individual child. They require more guesswork, and thoughtful consideration. Here are some.

Cigarette smoke. Cigarette smoke is an irritant that causes injury to a child's airway in ways other than the allergic pathway (tobacco is not much of an allergen). Irritants can cause a lot of harm. Oodles of data support that cigarette smoke is bad for children with "asthma." Admittedly, the studies don't break down the different types of asthma to determine if cigarette smoke is bad for some types of asthma and not others. However, my experience suggests (rather strongly) that cigarette smoke is pretty darn bad across the board. There are indeed children whose sole cause of asthma is the exposure to cigarette smoke. Chronic exposure to cigarette smoke in children with asthma can lead to permanent nonreversible airflow obstruction (sometimes called *remodeling*).

Chronic injury to the airway can lead to persistent and undesirable changes to tissues of the airway and to the way the airway functions. *Remodeling* is a term used to describe a bunch of changes that occur in the airways of children with chronic or recurrent airway injuries. Chronic injuries to the airway, from untreated allergic inflammation or exposures to irritants like cigarette smoke, can lead to scar-tissue accumulation around the airways, along with persistently increased gland size and mucus production within the airways. Scar formation can make the involved airways permanently (irreversibly) narrowed. The scarring is caused by the same processes that caused the asthma earlier. The scarring or remodeling is evident in spirometry (lung-function testing). One way to think of this scarring is that it takes a normal airway diameter and makes it narrower than average. And already narrower airways are more likely to become symptomatic when mucus accumulates, when bronchospasm happens, or when inflammatory swelling occurs. Basically, remodeling and the other changes from chronic airway injury increase the severity and chronicity of asthma.

In my opinion, children should not be exposed to cigarette smoke. And certainly children with asthma, regardless of the age or type of asthma, should not be exposed. Sure a whiff here or there is fine. Children aren't *allergic* to cigarette smoke, and won't have a dangerous immunologic response (such as can occur with food allergies). But cigarette smoke *is* a toxin—a poison to the cells of the airway and an irritant to the airway nerves. It hinders cilia cells from clearing mucus. It increases mucus production.

There is little to be said that is positive about cigarette smoke. If your child has asthma and you smoke cigarettes, what should you do?

There is no stronger motivation to quit than having a child with lung disease. Okay, it isn't easy to quit smoking. It is one of the hardest things a person can do. But you have to quit. There are no ifs ands or butts about that. You must quit smoking.

But, everyone is an individual and everyone is different. If you are filled with acute new stresses in your life, or fighting some other addiction (something more dangerous to your child's overall well-being like alcohol or heroin), then you may have to postpone the effort to quit smoking.

I hesitate to add that while you are quitting, you should not ever smoke in the car with your child present in it (even with the window cracked) and you must never smoke inside your house, whether your child is there or not. You should only smoke outdoors, even in the freezing rain and hot summer sweat.

Wood stoves. I suppose cigarette smokers say smoking cigarettes is awesome. But they're deluded by the addiction. Wood stoves, in contrast, really *are* awesome. There is little more wonderful than the warmth pouring out of a wood stove on a cold winter evening, knowing that the heat is fueled not by expensive oil or propane or electricity, but by dead trees. Nothing more awesome...

But...

Wood stoves can pump out smoke into the house. Every now and then there is a downdraft through the stovepipe when the draft isn't strong enough or the fire not hot enough. Windy days can reverse the flow intermittently down the chimney. Puffs of smoke can pour out the vents into the house.

What to do about wood stoves? This is a challenge. First, do whatever you can to make the stove work well. Ask experts in wood stove use (online discussion forums are great) to help make sure the smoke comes into the house as little as possible. Use well-seasoned wood (not just wood that the seller *claims* is well seasoned), because it will burn hotter and keep the draft stronger. You may need to raise the height of the chimney to improve draft and prevent downdrafts.

Is the wood stove the primary source of heat for the house? Then you may be stuck. If it is just a wonderfully enjoyable source of heat, but you have other options, then consider not using it until your child's asthma is very clearly under control, with essentially no asthma symptoms. Perhaps your child needs to be on good medicine that controls other types of asthma, or perhaps he needs a couple of years to outgrow small or malacic infant airways. When your child is totally fine, start using the wood stove again and see if he starts getting sick again. If not, great. If he gets sick, perhaps put the stove to rest for a few years before trying again.

The same thoughts are true for any heating source that dumps smoke into the house.

By the way, don't forget to make sure your carbon monoxide alarms are working.

Unusual stuff. I suggest you let your doctor know if there are special hobbies or crafts undertaken in your house, or less common pets or exposures, or lots of exposure to chlorinated pools. Anything that raises unusual types of dust or with strong chemicals released on a regular basis is worth telling your child's doctor about. Many unusual exposures cause diseases that don't involve the asthma process, but nonetheless can be confused. It is wise to tell your doctor about birds in the house, woodworking with certain types of wood, even playing brass musical instruments. There are many unusual causes of unusual diseases of the lung. These *hypersensitivity pneumonitis* diseases are caused by specific bacteria and molds, and don't look exactly (or even much) like asthma. They are rarely found in children and therefore not often considered by doctors other than allergists and pulmonologists. Let your doctor know about the unusual things in the environment in which you live.

Exercise

I would like to take this moment to discuss another important component of therapy for many children with asthma, and that is *exercise*. There is great *value* in exercise for *treating* children who tend to develop asthmatic symptoms.

Exercise has been shown to be more important than diet and weight loss to protect against the harmful effects of obesity. Exercise in asthmatic children is very often helpful whether they are obese or not. We don't yet have a grasp on which causes of asthma exercise is most helpful for.

Exercise stretches airway muscles through deep breathing. This may help prevent bronchospasm. Exercise improves cellular metabolic efficiency and may help reduce oxidative injury to cells (oxidative stress). Exercise may reduce the inflammation associated with obesity and allergies. Exercise has lots of valuable features.

It is true that exercise can trigger bronchospasm by drying the airway lining fluid. That response, however, can easily be prevented, leaving the benefits of exercise available. As a caveat, exercise during exacerbations of asthma is not a good idea. Your child should rest during active asthma exacerbations. But regular fun exercise is often a very good way to help *prevent* asthma from acting up. You will need to figure out how helpful it is for your own child, based on what you observe in him.

Almost assuredly, watching television is not helpful for children. They sit there, barely breathing, never taking deep sighing breaths, never stretching their airway muscles, all while passively absorbing propaganda that pours forth from the screen. Video games are probably better. But getting your child outside and active is likely to be better still. You need to decide along with your child what makes the most sense for him.

Now it is time to move on to the medications used for the various different causes of asthma.

CHAPTER 26

Getting Ready to Discuss Medications

One of the problems with the newfangled definition of asthma (the one that I don't like) and the way of thinking about asthma these days as if it were all one disease when it clearly is not, is that our knowledge about asthma medications has gotten all befuddled.

Pharmaceutical companies and academic scientists study medication effects in people with "asthma" without differentiating the underlying diseases, and then try to make conclusions. This makes as much sense to me as lumping all people with diarrhea into a single group and trying a single medication on them to see if it works. It may work in some with one diarrheal disease, and not in others with a different diarrheal disease, and the data will be a mess and the study shockingly unhelpful. That is how I feel most asthma medication studies are these days: expensive and unhelpful.

Because of this, lots of the data in the last couple of decades are worthy of the trash bin, not the medical textbook.

I try to sort through what works and what doesn't seem to work *in general*.

But your child is special and unique, of course, and generalities are only useful to guide us. For all the hassles of asthma, we are fortunate about one thing, which is that it takes little time to see if an intervention we try is helpful in an individual patient. It might take as little as a day or a month to see the results of an intervention. It is not something we have to wait years to see effects of. And if we try something that doesn't work

159

(common) or that even makes asthma worse in your child (uncommon), we can stop it and move to something else.

In other words, we can use the empiric-trial methodology beyond just the diagnostic empiric trial. We can try different things, guided by (but not enslaved or restricted by) what has worked in other children and other settings, and see what combinations and tricks work best for your child with the type(s) of asthma that he has. And this can be done with little risk.

Asthma is not cancer. In cancer, the doctors can't try one thing and then another and another, because the cancer doesn't give them that luxury. So the doctors have to hope that the way other children with cancer responded to a given medical regimen will be a good guide for how this new child with cancer will do on that therapy. They have to rely on evidence-based medicine (average data from studies) because that is all they have available to guide them. They hope it gives them good guidance to select wisely the therapeutic regimen for a child with recently diagnosed cancer.

Fortunately for us, asthma is entirely unlike cancer. Unless the asthma is exacerbated right now, it gives us the luxury of trying different regimens of therapies to see how they work to keep asthma under control in *your* child. We have the luxury of trying all sorts of ideas if we want to, smartly and sanely. If the asthma is not responding to one therapy well, we can quickly change course.

Because of this, I don't disdain efforts at safe alternative sorts of therapy for asthma. If you get interested in an herbal remedy, and want to give it a try, then as long as you have researched it, trust the practitioner who recommends it, and don't lie to yourself about it, then I am all in favor of trying it. I can't advise you about the alternative sorts of therapies like naturopaths and herbalists can, because I don't have their training and experience. Nor can I advise you about potential nutritional interventions that some say help with "asthma." But I can advise you to always be rational about the process; keep the emotions, the hype, and the pathologic hopefulness out of your thinking, and be logical. I advise you the same way when it comes to the standard pharma-company drugs that I do know a whole lot about. There is certainly hype and lies and misleading statements and advertising in this realm too. Stay rational and thoughtful. And remember that if someone claims they have the ultimate, best treatment/cure for asthma, ask them what *type* of asthma they are so good at treating. If your question throws them off and they don't even know what you mean, then what they offer (although possibly still of some value) is groupthinky and probably not well thought out.

As you try different interventions for your child's asthma, if something doesn't work and it has been given a good and *smart* try, then move on to something else. Test interventions by means of empiric trials, which means putting some effort into measuring or comparing how your child is doing before and after the intervention.

One other thought. Asthma is caused by multiple different disorders that can overlap. Some of the disorders, such as allergic airway inflammation, in turn involve hundreds of biochemical pathways. It is therefore acceptable and even wise to be prepared to use several medications for your child's asthma all at once. This is not the sort of "polypharmacy" that should cause you to be fearful. Not at all. Rather it is smart to treat the diseases that underlie your child's asthma and it may take 3 or 4 or even 5 medications to do so, at least some of the time. That sounds horrible, but don't be horrified. It is just fine. Here's why: the asthma medications are almost all really safe.

But the medications can be expensive, and that is troublesome...

Generic medications are fine. Less expensive medications are fine. I will discuss these cheaper options soon.

The next chapter focuses on drug therapy for the biggest problem for most asthma:

If you have a high deductible or no health insurance and want to get prescription medications for as low a personal cost as if your health insurance covered them, look at www.GoodRx.com. It is a free and excellent service that provides coupons for your local and national pharmacies that reduces the prices of medications by 80% or more. It is the free market trying to work in a system in which there is otherwise hardly any free market left to help you. I cannot encourage you strongly enough to check it out. It is an exceptional website.

inflammation. But first let's take a moment to discuss how to use medications that are useful for asthma.

Medications you might use for asthma come in several forms:

- *Oral* (for swallowing), as pills or liquid or soluble tablets or powders
- *Inhaled*
  - Via a metered-dose inhaler (MDI) from a pressurized canister, possibly with a *spacer*
  - Via a dry-powder inhalation device (DPI), with no spacer
  - Via a nebulizer machine that makes an inhalable mist from a liquid medicine
- *Injection* is used by clinics and hospitals.

Swallowing pills and liquids is straightforward.

But inhalation of medications is best accomplished using some simple tricks, and the tricks differ depending on the inhalation device used.

A metered dose inhaler (MDI) is a pressurized canister that your child (or you) needs to press down on (actuate) to release some medication in a puff of mist, and that mist is supposed to be inhaled. Important—*shake* the MDI just before each actuation! A *spacer* device is a tube or an accordion device that will have a small volume of air in it that the mist gets squirted into first. Many of these *spacers* have clear walls so you can see the medicine inside. This spacer should have a mask attached to it for use in infants and smaller children, or a mouthpiece for older children who are able to cooperate more fully. After actuating the MDI into the spacer, your child needs to slowly breathe the medication in from the spacer. See Figure 6.

The point of the spacer device is twofold. First, the medication as it comes out of the MDI device is in tiny (but visible) droplets that consist of a mixture of the medication and a rapidly evaporating propellant. When these droplets are visible, that means they are too big to inhale effectively into the lungs, because momentum causes most of the medication droplets to just smash into the back of the throat. Essentially, visible droplets (although tiny) have too much momentum to turn the corner in the back of the throat to go down through the larynx. Inside the spacer device, however, there is a second or two for the propellant to evaporate out of the droplets into gas phase. Then the medication droplets get so small that you can't see them anymore. They're still there, but they

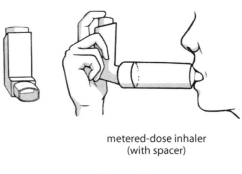

metered-dose inhaler
(with spacer)

Figure 6

are now small enough that they can turn corners better during inhalation, and can get into your child's lungs. So you see, you want your child actually to inhale *invisible* medication!

The second purpose of the spacer is to make it easier for your child to coordinate the breathing of the medication. Puff the medication into the spacer, count to 2 or 3 seconds, and then have your child inhale slowly.

A spacer is almost always valuable to use with an MDI.

Dry-powder inhalers (DPI) work differently. They are not pressurized. You do not use a spacer with them. The medication has no propellant, but is simply a fine powder. The powder is sucked into your child's airways when he inhales hard. So, in contrast to the slow breath used for an MDI, your child has to suck fast and hard on a DPI. They are generally used in children over age 5 years who can suck in hard enough. See Figure 7.

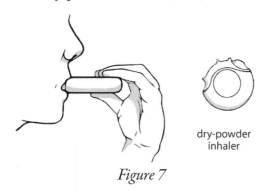

dry-powder
inhaler

Figure 7

Nebulizers provide a mist of medication that a child can breathe for several minutes through a mouthpiece, or through a mask, or just out of

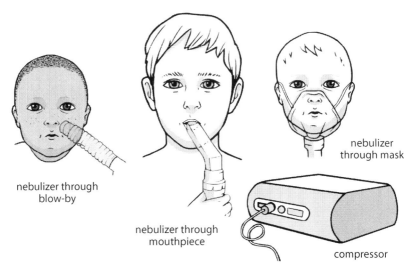

nebulizer through
blow-by

nebulizer through
mouthpiece

nebulizer
through mask

compressor

Figure 8

the air ("blow-by") from a tube near her nose or mouth. These devices are well known to most with asthmatic children. They take longer to give each dose than is required for a DPI or MDI, but nebulizers are useful at any age. See Figure 8.

For all devices, the amount of medication that actually gets to the airways of the chest is highly variable, from 0% of the listed dose if used improperly, to 5–15% in most methods, to occasionally as high as 50% in some of the newer MDIs. In your child, we don't know what percentage of the drug will actually be delivered to the airway. All we can do is make sure that the device is used properly so that the drug is not wasted, and then treat your child like the individual that he is by providing whatever dose seems to work for him, while following how he does with care and love.

For all the studies of how much drug gets delivered from each device, one thing is clear—it is dependent on the patient. With the huge variation in deposition of medicine in the lung from person to person, it makes sense to be very flexible with dosing, always seeking what works to help the individual child feel better and stay healthy.

Keep in mind that children taking "high dose" inhaled medications may actually be getting a very low dose if the device they are using doesn't work well for them or they aren't using it correctly.

Also, here is a good place to mention that if your child is taking inhaled steroid medication, it is wise to have him rinse his mouth out after taking his puffs (MDI) or inhalations (DPI) or nebulization treatment. Although inhaled steroids are safe drugs, they can occasionally lead to thrush in the mouth (yeast infection). Rinsing the mouth or brushing teeth after taking inhaled steroids works well to prevent that from happening. In infants and small children who haven't figured out the "rinse and spit" concept, just have them drink something after a treatment.

CHAPTER 27

Symptomatic Therapy for Asthma

Treating the symptoms of asthma is usually the least important part of asthma management in the *long* run, but doing so is important in the *short* run because we want our children to feel better when they are sick. And indeed, treating the acute symptoms of a bad asthma exacerbation may be critically necessary to assure good oxygen is getting through the lungs and into the blood. Now *that's* important!

I prefer to focus on *prevention* of exacerbations of asthma whenever possible, so that the children don't get sick much at all. But asthma exacerbations do happen sometimes despite all our best efforts. Symptomatic therapy is important to have available and to know about. It is valuable to have created with your child's doctor an *asthma action plan* that is written specifically for your child and based on your child's asthma diagnoses and history. This written action plan will help remind you of what to do in the event of an asthma exacerbation, especially if you are prone to be panicky.

Bronchoconstriction can happen in seconds to minutes, and it can be reversed with medication almost as fast. Because of this, bronchodilation drugs that reverse bronchoconstriction are a mainstay of symptomatic therapy. They are also the most well-known drugs for asthma. This does *not* mean they are the *best* drugs for asthma, though. The best drugs *prevent* asthma episodes. Except in the case of exercise-induced asthma, the bronchodilator drugs do very little to prevent asthma episodes from happening.

The bronchodilator drugs don't always work to treat an acute exacerbation. Bronchoconstriction is, after all, but one of many causes of airflow limitation. The fact that bronchoconstriction is *an* important cause of airflow obstruction and that the drugs generally work *fast* is what makes them a mainstay of therapy.

The most common bronchodilator drug is albuterol (called "salbutamol" in Europe). It is in a class of drugs called *beta2-agonists* that work to relax the muscle surrounding the airways. There are a bunch of different beta2-agonists for sale these days. They can be taken orally, injected, or inhaled (by nebulizer or MDI or DPI), but overwhelmingly nowadays we use the inhaled versions of bronchodilators. Some bronchodilators are considered "short acting," like albuterol (which starts working within minutes and lasts for a few hours), and some are "long acting," which usually take a bit longer to start working but may last for 12 hours or more.

Of course, I recommend following the directions of your doctor in regard to the use of beta2-agonists (such as albuterol).

Remember that each child interacts differently with any given device for inhaled medication (MDI, DPI, or nebulizer). It is uncertain therefore how much of an inhaled medication your child might need to take at any given juncture. Fortunately, the short-acting medications start working quickly enough that you can see whether they are working or not. The side effects of them (increased heart rate, shakiness) also appear rapidly. Using your home fingertip oxygen saturation monitor, you can follow your child's pulse rate and see how much of the medication is getting absorbed. Within fifteen minutes of inhaling albuterol, his heart rate should rise. For example, it might rise 10-50% faster than his normal heart rate. That is safe in almost every child, just like it is safe for the heart rate to double with exercise. (But in older adults, this speeding up of the heart rate too far can be more dangerous.)

Within a few minutes, you should notice a bronchodilator medication like albuterol begin to work (increasing heart rate a bit and breathing easier), and within 30 minutes you should see that dose's maximal effect (from that one dose) and be able to decide if you can and should give another dose to your child (if you want to see if there will be more effect). If, after the first dose of albuterol, your child still has troublesome symptoms of bad wheezing or difficulty breathing, then giving additional doses soon is wise. Get help from a doctor until you are confident in what you are doing.

Beta2-agonists are important drugs for symptomatic improvement for allergic inflammatory asthma, viral-triggering of allergic inflammatory asthma, exercise-induced asthma, viral-induced asthma, and to a lesser extent in some of the irritant-induced asthma (chlorine).

Beta2-agonists are sometimes useful in viral bronchiolitis, but often do little good because viral bronchiolitis involves more secretions and inflammation rather than bronchospasm. But again, in the viral-induced asthma that comes with subsequent common cold infections in the months to years *after* bronchiolitis, beta2-agonists are usually helpful.

However, it is important to keep in mind that these bronchodilator drugs, for the most part, are symptomatic therapy only. They do little for the underlying problems that caused the bronchospasm in the first place. These drugs do not block allergic inflammation. These drugs do not stop viral infections. Also, these drugs do little to counter the excess mucous gland production. Furthermore beta2-agonists sometimes can over-relax airways with malacia, making malacia symptomatically worse.

The *long-acting* bronchodilators (such as salmeterol—one of the components of Advair) take a bit longer to start working and aren't therefore as often used for rapid treatment of acute bronchospasm. They are used in adults to try to keep the bronchi relaxed. The long-acting beta-agonists (which are called LABA) are used for maintenance therapy and prevention of symptoms. I personally don't prescribe long-acting bronchodilators very often in children, but I am not necessarily in the majority of pediatricians in this regard.

The short-acting beta2-agonists such as albuterol are important to use to help your child get through an asthma exacerbation. They can help open up airways so that your child doesn't get sicker. They can keep the lungs sufficiently open to keep good oxygen getting to the blood. They can give the anti-inflammatory drugs time to kick in to treat allergic inflammation, or provide time for the virus to pass. So these rapid-acting drugs are important.

The only times I prescribe long-acting beta2-agonists are under two conditions:

1. When I think that bronchospasm is a child's sole cause of asthma, such as in many children who have only exercise-induced asthma;

2. When despite maximal efforts at controlling underlying inflammation, and after I have exhaustively searched for other causes of asthma, there are still symptoms of asthma present that respond to bronchodilator therapy.

One of the reasons I try to avoid using long-acting bronchodilators as a therapy for asthma is that, outside of exercise-induced asthma, the symptoms of asthma (such as cough and wheeze) are one of the best indicators of there being a persistent disease process in the airway that is not being adequately treated. This might be undertreated inflammation of some kind. Remember, we don't have much ability to measure airway inflammation. Therefore we rely on symptoms as an indicator of the presence of a disease, and we lose that indicator if we treat those symptoms while leaving the underlying disease unaddressed. It is like taking morphine to take away the pain of appendicitis and thereby hoping (dangerously) to skip the surgery. Often symptoms are there to tell us something is wrong. Covering them up, instead of treating what underlies them, can be a mistake.

Although the short-acting beta-agonists are just treating symptoms too, they are used primarily when there *are active symptoms*. But long acting beta-agonists are marketed for use regularly, every day, for the purpose of *blocking* symptoms and are supposed to be used whether the symptoms are present or not. You can see that with regular use of long acting beta-agonists, we lose the symptom signal that should be there to tell us that the underlying disease is not controlled.

There are times when inhaled beta2-agonists like albuterol don't work, even when bronchoconstriction is quite active. You see, albuterol is supposed to get to the bronchoconstricting muscle that surrounds an airway by crossing through the wall of the airway from the inside, and that means that the medication needs to be able to get to that location. But airways that are obstructed (by mucus and severe inflammatory swelling, for example) block the access of the inhaled medicine to the airways beyond. Also, if the airways are acidic, most beta2-agonists (including albuterol) have trouble getting through the airway wall, and so can't relax the bronchoconstricting muscles as well. A child who has an acute wheezing episode and shortness of breath and in whom drugs like albuterol don't work needs aggressive therapy directed against whatever is causing her asthma. In some types of asthma, the passage of time is the most important therapy, but sometimes that time has to pass while a child is in the hospital.

There are other rapid-acting bronchodilator drugs that are occasionally used in childhood asthma.

Inhaled anticholinergic medications are airway muscle relaxers that work in children, although they have never taken the place of albuterol, probably because albuterol has been the most commonly used drug for a long time. Medicine has momentum. It is hard for a new drug to push albuterol aside. These inhaled anticholinergic medications do have some advantages that you and your doctor may want to consider. In some children they can decrease glandular secretion, and that may be useful in those children in whom secretions are a big cause of airflow obstruction. (These anticholinergic drugs might possibly thicken mucus, though, which isn't good.) There are also some doctors who think that these drugs cause less trouble than the beta2-agonists do for children with malacia.

Anticholinergics may be excellent medications to help treat acute symptoms in your child. The only way to know is to give them a try here and there, and see for yourself. Check with your child's doctor. You can get a combination of albuterol and ipratropium (the most common inhaled anticholinergic) in a nebulizer (brand name Duoneb) and thus have two different bronchodilators together. Or you can just mix together one dose of ipratropium and one dose of albuterol in a nebulizer solution yourself, for a lot cheaper. Sometimes the combination works best.

It's okay to try different things, and even repeat trials from time to time, to see what seems to work for your child. That's the great thing about asthma and bronchodilators. You can really make progress personalizing your child's asthma care by getting essentially immediate feedback about how the medications seem to work. It is definitely possible to overdose though, so make sure to discuss the medication plans with your doctor.

If a stuffy nose triggers asthma-like symptoms in your child, *keeping the nose clear* can provide remarkable help in treating the acute asthma. Saline (salt water) drops in the nose followed by suction can help in infants. Also, under the advice of your doctor, decongestants can be used, including infrequent use of topical decongestants. These decongestant drugs are not recommended by pediatricians much anymore, but that is because they don't help much in otherwise healthy children with colds, and there are some side effects. I am glad they aren't recommended for colds *in general,* but they still have a role for children whose colds result in lots of problems with narrowing and obstruction of airways in the chest. Such children are not "otherwise healthy," because they get breathing difficulty with colds, and that changes the whole risk/reward assessment of decongestants. The decongestant drugs can be tried in children with asthma and some children with malacia, but keep your doctor in the loop.

Acetaminophen (Tylenol) and ibuprofen are also useful symptomatic therapy in children with fevers in whom *relative airway narrowing* becomes apparent because of the greater amount of air they need to move through their lungs during the high metabolism of a fever. Children with smaller or already-narrowed airways may well become symptomatic with wheezing and difficulty breathing during the fever as their airflow becomes turbulent. Knocking down the fever can help them feel better and breathe more easily. The same is true for a child with any cause of asthma: fever increases a child's need to move air. Fever should be treated so that the child can breathe easier.

I want to reiterate that taking beta2-agonists like albuterol can make children feel better with asthma, but this class of medications does nothing to improve any inflammation that may underlie the asthma. Again, I don't think it is wise to cover up ongoing signs of disease by using symptomatic therapy alone. It's kinda like painting over rotten wood in the hull of a boat and lying to yourself that the craft then won't sink.

And when it comes to allergic inflammatory asthma, the need for frequent use of bronchodilator medications to treat symptoms is usually a very good indicator that inflammation needs more aggressive intervention of some kind: perhaps a different medication regimen, or better environmental control, or reconsideration of the diagnosis.

For allergic inflammatory asthma, I aim to assure that children are healthy enough that they need to use albuterol less than a couple of times per week. That's pretty good control.

For viral-induced asthma, I recommend using albuterol whenever it is needed and only when it is needed (with wheezing from colds), but perhaps throw in some montelukast as well (see next chapter).

All of the above information can help you to craft, with your child's doctor, an asthma action plan that is tailored to your child's needs. So please do create such a plan and get it on paper.

Then don't lose the paper!

CHAPTER 28

Medications for Allergic Inflammation and Allergic Inflammatory Asthma

There are many types of inflammation. And there are different types of medications that treat airway inflammation. Some of these medications have been available for many decades but, because of the distortions of the health insurance system and the FDA, remain moderately expensive in the United States. There are new medications (that are almost invariably *ridiculously* expensive) that target particular aspects of inflammation, including some focused on allergic inflammation, and these drugs can be helpful in various illnesses.

Despite the expense of the medication, inflammation is important to treat if it is present, and if it is possible to treat it, which it sometimes isn't. Fortunately, allergic inflammation is usually treatable. Viral inflammation is a whole lot less treatable.

I divide the treatments based on the asthma diagnosis. You know that the underlying diagnoses can overlap some; thus appropriate treatment may involve intelligent combinations of the various medications.

Let's start with *therapy for allergic inflammatory asthma*. (I will discuss therapy for other asthma diagnoses in the next chapters.)

Inhaled Steroid Medication

The most successful medication type for treatment of allergic inflammatory asthma in most children is *inhaled steroid medication.*

175

But of course that doesn't mean that inhaled steroids will work for *your* child. It depends on the diagnoses and on your child.

Inhaled steroids take a day or more to begin working in asthma, so they are *not* drugs that are used *alone* in the treatment of an acute active "asthma attack" when a child is having lots of trouble breathing. Please make sure you realize this. Inhaled steroids don't work fast to lessen symptoms.

Inhaled steroids can be used every day (or less often) to treat and prevent allergic-inflammatory asthma and its symptoms, or they can be used seasonally, or used in pulses alongside other medications for the treatment of acute exacerbations.

I would like to calm fears you may have about inhaled steroids. The type of steroids we use for asthma diagnosis and therapy has nothing to do with body building. It's different stuff altogether. And inhaled steroids are used in pretty darn low doses too. They are not completely free of side effects, but they are remarkably safe. As with all medications, we don't want to use them if they don't do any good, and we want to use them (in the long run) at the lowest effective dose. But I trust inhaled steroids.

The first step is to see if they work in *your child* as well as they work in the average child with asthma symptoms.

The asthma guidelines that most doctors were trained to follow lump all kids with asthma together, because "asthma" is considered a diagnosis. Doctors have been taught (I believe incorrectly) to initially prescribe a *low* dose of inhaled steroid in children with "asthma" and over time increase the dosing until the child is better.

That would be okay if you *knew* that your child had airway inflammation that was going to respond to a sufficient dose of inhaled steroid. But the reality is that you actually *don't* know that your child has this type of airway inflammation, and you don't know what a sufficient dose of medication for *your* child would be if he has that type of inflammation! And the doctors don't know either.

In the usually recommended "start low" regimen, your child may well have continued asthma symptoms either because the dosage is too low or because inhaled steroids aren't ever going to do the trick for him.

To avoid this delay in getting your child well, you may need to suggest to your doctor a different strategy than the expert guidelines put forth.

What I suggest is a diagnostic empiric trial. An empiric trial of inhaled steroids is a diagnostic test, not a therapy, that may help you sort this out. Please see chapter 10, in which is presented the *diagnostic empiric trial,* for more details. This is not a lifetime treatment. It is just a test to see if inhaled steroids are likely to work in your child.

As one example of a diagnostic empiric trial, I use *high-dose* inhaled steroids initially. I recommend high dose for a period of only a few weeks and see if the asthma is markedly improved. If it is effective, that means that your child probably has airway inflammation that responds to steroids. If your child is not better at all, then steroid-responsive asthma is far less likely, and you have learned that information quickly. I want to reiterate that allergic inflammatory asthma is usually highly responsive to inhaled steroids.

Steroid comes in inhaled versions (of multiple different doses, brands, and drugs). Steroid medication also comes as an oral (swallowed) form that is used to treat significant exacerbations of asthma, and which has side effects that are not desirable, but sometimes necessary to accept. And steroids can be given by injection (used in a clinic, emergency room, or hospital).

When there is suspicion of two or more concurrent causes of asthma in a child who has been suffering with it for too long, and when parents are sick of the whole thing, it is often helpful to try several empiric trials (different medications) all at once in the hope of *capturing health.* I will tell you how I might do that in a little bit after I discuss a few other medications.

The key point is that diagnostic empiric trials of medications are not "trial and error" medicine, not by any means. Instead, a trial of a medication is one of the best types of diagnostic test in asthma, and one, two, or five such trials with different medications or combinations is totally acceptable. These trials help us personalize the care for your child and your child's specific type(s) of asthma.

As I mentioned, the steroid medications work very well for treatment of *allergic inflammatory asthma.* Allergic inflammatory asthma is asthma that arises because of allergic reactions to stuff that your child inhales. It is the most common type of asthma. It tends to occur more in late preschool years and school-age children, because it takes a few years of living before allergies to inhaled stuff can develop.

So, if your child has *allergic inflammatory asthma*, meaning he has asthma and tests positive for relevant allergens like dust mite, cat, pollen, etc., then the first and most important drug class for the treatment of your child is likely to be inhaled steroid. The medical literature and experience tell us this. Now we need to show that it works in your child.

If your child's history makes it seem that allergic inflammatory asthma is the only asthma diagnosis she has (with or without viral-triggering), then you can proceed to an empiric trial of inhaled steroids, at high dose, for a month perhaps, and see what happens.

If there is clearly an excellent response, meaning a clear reduction or elimination of asthma symptoms, and improvement in lung-function scores, then you have successfully used the diagnostic empiric trial to confirm that steroid-responsive allergic inflammation underlies your child's asthma. And you have proven within a reasonable doubt that inhaled steroids are an effective medication for *your* child's asthma. And that is so much more useful information than knowing that 70% got better out of some group of kids studied at the National Institutes of Health. You now *know* that inhaled steroids work in *your* child's asthma.

Now, with the diagnosis confirmed and an effective therapy in hand, you have a drug in your armamentarium against asthma that you have seen work in *your* child, that is *proven* in your child to work. It is likely that the inhaled steroids will become your best method to keep your child's inflammation—and therefore his asthma—under control. But it will also be time to lower the dose of the inhaled steroids to the lowest effective dose. As you lower the dose, you watch your child to see if the asthma starts appearing or getting more troublesome. As you lower the dose periodically (perhaps each week), you can see if everything is okay. If not, raise the dose again for a while.

Each child is different and best dosing adjustments can't be predicted. But, I will often recommend halving the dose from the diagnostic empiric trial and see how that goes for a couple of weeks, and if all is well, halving it again. Then work down slowly after that.

If however, the diagnostic empiric trial of high-dose inhaled steroids yielded no evidence of benefit—meaning your child did not get better—then some more thought is required to figure out what's up. At least it didn't take six months of slowly raising the dose to figure out that we were on the wrong track! *Vive la* diagnostic empiric trial!

The first thing I do if a child is not getting better on inhaled steroids is to make sure that the child is using the medication correctly, at the intended high dose. Sometimes (actually pretty often), children and parents forget how to use the inhaled medications, and then the medicine doesn't get to where it is supposed to get (the airways of the chest), in which case the diagnostic empiric trial could have failed not because inhaled steroids won't work for your child, but because we have to find a better version of the medicine for your child or fix the way he is taking it.

Second, you and your doctor need to think together about whether there was some other change that made the asthma a lot worse during this time, such as catching the cold or the flu, or a huge exposure to a cat that he didn't have when you started the trial. In other words, is it possible he failed to get better during the diagnostic empiric trial because without the medication he would have gotten a whole lot worse? Perhaps the inhaled steroid prevented such worsening, but wasn't adequate to make him *better* during that stress. These events are possible and confusing and may require a repeat effort at the diagnostic empiric trial later.

Third, the working diagnosis for your child's asthma may not be correct, or may not be complete. Were we wrong about the allergy tests? Did they lie to us? Or is he allergic, yes, but not getting exposed to the allergens to which he is allergic and therefore they are irrelevant, leaving us needing to look for another cause? Might your child have acid reflux as a contributor? Could she have some inhalational toxin exposure that we didn't think of (like cigarette exposure)? Could there be a component or a dominance

A "working diagnosis" is a diagnosis that is not confirmed, but your doctor thinks is likely and often gets confirmed by means of a successful diagnostic empiric trial.

The term "steroid-resis-tant asthma" has been used a lot and is perhaps an okay subcategory of asthma (but is not a diag-nosis). Asthma may be steroid resistant because the asthma is caused by something other than inflammation, or caused by a type of inflamma-tion that we know never improves with steroids, or because the steroid medi-cations aren't taken cor-rectly, or because there are too many confound-ing concurrent diagno-ses left unrecognized and untreated, *or* because the child has a missing cel-lular receptor for the ste-roids (so that there is no way they could work). If we expect steroids to work for a child's asthma, and they don't, then it is important to seek a precise reason why they failed.

of vocal cord syndrome? These other causes and confounders of asthma aren't expected to improve with inhaled steroids. In other words, if the diagnostic empiric trial failed, well, it is time to start looking for other diagnoses that may be contributing to your child's asthma.

It's all part of the diagnostic process. Remember, a diagnostic empiric trial of inhaled steroids is a *test* to see if there is steroid-responsive inflammation (usually allergic) *in your child*.

Fourth, there are some, *very rare*, children who have the same inflammation as other allergic asthmatic children, but who don't respond to inhaled steroids because they don't have a normally functioning cellular receptor for the steroids.

Let's go back to the case in which your child's asthma clearly responds well to inhaled steroids. I would like to introduce you to another reality of asthma management that is particularly relevant for allergic inflammatory asthma. It is this: because the disease changes over time (getting worse and better as allergen exposures increase or decrease and as cold viruses infect your child) you should be prepared to change the dose of inhaled steroids pretty frequently.

When your child is not in his allergy season, you may be able to cut the inhaled steroid dosing down the most. I usually don't entirely stop inhaled steroids in children with allergic inflammatory asthma, but in children whose asthma is completely under control (no symptoms at all), I may wean them down to as little as one puff (one dose) once a week. Yep, only once a week. It's but a tiny whiff of steroid, but remember that those allergy cells in the airway are very sensitive to steroids, and so one dose once a week can be enough. It might be enough for your child, or your child might need a lot more.

Then, just before a relevant allergy season begins, I will recommend increasing the inhaled steroids to shoot for at least a modest dose daily, to try to prevent inhaled allergens from causing significant inflammation. (I may also add other medications depending on your child's history, to help prevent and control the inflammation.)

If your child has viral-triggering of his allergic inflammatory asthma, then I recommend increasing the dose of inhaled steroids to high and even very high doses at the onset of any cold, and that means as soon as you *think* a cold might be present. This might triple or quadruple your child's normal dose, or even much more if he had been on a low once-a-week dose. Now, this really big increase in steroid dosing, too, is an empiric trial. It won't work in all children. It is designed to see if this increase in inhaled steroid dosage at the onset of colds seems to protect your child from the viral-triggered exacerbations. If it does seem to protect your child, great. If it doesn't seem to protect your child, then we can probably put that intervention aside (not use it) and should move on to try other interventions (see the section below on leukotriene modifiers).

Sadly, at the time of writing (and historically too), cheap pricing has not emerged for inhaled steroids in the United States. There are many different inhaled steroids to choose among, sold by different pharmaceutical companies. They are all effective, they have different doses, and different metabolisms by the liver, and cost somewhat different amounts (all expensive). Does it matter what inhaled steroid you choose?

Here's my view on choosing inhaled steroids.

As I mentioned before, medication inhaled from a puffer or a dry-powder inhaler or from a nebulizer (the devices from which most inhaled medications are dispensed) doesn't all get into the airways of the chest. Actually, the majority of the medication released by these devices goes out into the atmosphere, the next-largest fraction lands in the mouth and pharynx to be swallowed, and only a minority goes to the chest airways and lungs. The percentage that goes into the chest airways (the target of their action) ranges enormously from child to child and from device to device.

The devices used to deliver inhaled medications involve very complex regulatory scrutiny by FDA to confirm that they squirt out precisely the same dose each time. And indeed the devices do a good job of squirting out the same amount of drug each time. But children are not (yet) subject to the scrutiny of FDA. The inhalation maneuver is performed so differently from child to child that the device's functional delivery is really but a small issue. FDA nonetheless demands that devices obey their expensive precision rules, and this has kept the generic manufacturers out of the business. The lack of generic competition along with the fact that they are still prescription drugs (they should be over the counter!) are the main reasons why the prices for inhaled steroids remain high ($200/month or more).

In fact, there are some children who somehow manage to get no effective dose from a given device. When I see a child who is allergic and follows the pattern that makes me think he probably has allergic airway inflammation underlying his asthma but does *not* respond to inhaled steroids, then, in addition to thinking about all the potential other causes of asthma, I also consider that the drug might be failing because the child isn't using the device correctly, or the device and child don't work together well. It's not the child's fault, and not the device's fault. It is just a combination that doesn't work for the child. It is important for me to observe how the parent and child use the device to make sure that it at least *looks* like it is getting some medication into the lung.

There are older inhaled steroid medications that work just fine for allergic inflammatory asthma. And there are newer medications that work fine. Some of the inhaled steroids are more potent (stronger action per microgram) than others, but so what? The lower-potency drugs can just be used in higher dosage, and since they are lower potency, their side effects in general aren't any greater (all the inhaled steroids have low side effects, actually). Academic doctors and pharma folk argue over which inhaled steroid is better (in large group studies), but that is totally irrelevant to whether the drug works in your child or what dosage your child ends up needing. We should be constantly changing the dose up and down as your child needs it, and if the one your child uses has lower potency, you just end up using a higher dose. Potency and safety are inverses of each other (for the most part), so if you have a low-potency steroid, you have an inherently safer steroid, and vice versa.

Some of the newer medications have one advantage that may be worth caring about. I mentioned that much of the dose of inhaled steroid gets swallowed. The portion of drug that is swallowed isn't getting to the airway, but can go elsewhere in the body after being absorbed from the gut. The medication that is swallowed can go places you don't want it to go in the body. Fortunately, the liver is the first stop for almost everything that is swallowed into the gut, and the liver metabolizes away (cleans up and clears out) some of the swallowed steroid. Swallowed inhaled steroids get eliminated either partly, or entirely, by the liver, straight from the gut, *before* the drug gets to the rest of the body. The *newer* steroids tend to be nearly completely eliminated by the liver, and that seems a good thing. But it is not the ultimate, most important thing on the planet by any means.

> The issue of one inhaled steroid being "better" than another is what might now be called "a first-world problem." The reality is that they are all great medications, with exceedingly minor differences.

In the United States, at least, there is no rhyme or reason to the pricing of these drugs when insurance companies are involved. So, in my view, pick the cheapest of the drugs that undergo good liver metabolism. And if you find an older inhaled steroid that doesn't have as good liver metabolism but is a ton cheaper, that's going to be okay to use too.

If you have managed to avoid the manacles of health insurance and pay for your own medications directly, then you can get a bum deal a lot of the time in our current system in the United States. You can use generics when available. They are usually just fine and often tons cheaper. Also, use www.GoodRx.com to help you get prices that are much lower for most medications (although right now it doesn't help all that much with most inhaled medications). GoodRx.com costs you nothing to use, and seems to get for individuals the prices that the insurance companies negotiate from pharmacies, which are often small fractions of the usual cash price. Next, check out online pharmacies, often from Canada, where prices can be much lower and they will mail you your medications in a couple of weeks. There are nice Internet search engines that will help you find the cheapest prices.

There is one generic inhaled steroid in the United States right now, which is budesonide nebulizer solution (the generic version of Pulmicort). Because of the FDA, all the MDIs and DPIs are branded drugs, even though their patents have long expired. These drugs are cheap to make, but expensive to you because the FDA keeps competition off the market. Yes, that is kinda lame isn't it?

Overall I think the various inhaled steroids are all roughly equivalent in their usefulness and safety, although their doses are different because the steroids have different potency.

Leukotriene Modifiers

There is another class of anti-inflammatory medication that is useful in allergic inflammatory asthma. This type of drug was originally approved by the regulatory authorities for treatment of bronchoconstriction. But the anti-inflammatory properties are pretty good, and different from the anti-inflammatory properties of the inhaled steroids. This class is called "leukotriene modifiers," or "leukotriene antagonists."

I won't go into the scientific details of leukotriene pathways that contribute to asthma, but rather just summarize that the leukotrienes themselves are compounds that trigger bronchospasm and contribute to inflammation. Leukotrienes are released in the airway under various pathologic conditions, including in allergic asthma and in viral-induced asthma. Blocking them seems to cause no harm at all, so from that point of view, this class of drugs that block leukotrienes is mostly safe.

Leukotriene modifiers are designed as swallowed drugs, not inhaled drugs. They take hours or days to work. They are, for some children, exactly the right therapy for controlling their allergic inflammatory asthma, but in other children they seem to do nothing at all. Right now, we have no clinical way to determine in advance if the leukotriene pathway is playing a lead role in your child's asthma, so the only way to figure it out is to use a diagnostic empiric trial. In other words, try the medication and do your best to assess if it is working.

The most common leukotriene modifier used in children is montelukast, which came initially under the brand name Singulair. In the United States it is now available as an affordable generic, and at the time of writing the generic is about 6% of the cost of the brand. Yes, that is 6% of the brand cost! That's amazing! Montelukast (or Singulair if you feel like shelling out 15 times the money) may or may not work for your child. If it doesn't work in your child, put it aside.

It is common for me to start both an inhaled steroid at high dose *and* a leukotriene-modifying drug in a patient who I think has allergic inflammatory asthma. Then, assuming with this regimen that we "capture health" (basically get the asthma under complete control), we can cut out either the inhaled steroid or the leukotriene modifier and see what happens, and then start reducing the dosages to the minimum amount that seems to keep the asthma under control.

By the way, once you know the diagnosis with reasonable confidence, you can raise and lower the dosages of medications for various periods of time when your child needs them. Allergic inflammation increases with exposures and viral infections, and so the medications may well need to be raised (and later lowered) frequently. These dosage adjustments are usually based on symptoms and, when available, lung-function testing. But you can make dosage increases also when you *expect* trouble to arise, such as during your child's allergy season(s) or during peak seasons when the common cold appears in your community—or in your house.

The leukotriene-modifier drugs are intriguingly helpful for children who have viral-triggering of their allergic inflammatory asthma. In fact, for children with lots of viral-triggering of their allergic asthma, I prescribe montelukast frequently, especially during the times when the common colds are spreading among the community. And now that montelukast is pretty cheap, I expect I would prescribe it more. Always with the purpose of, first, just seeing if it will work in each child.

I will discuss montelukast again when I present therapy for viral-induced asthma.

Nasal Steroids

A key trigger for allergic inflammatory asthma is allergen inhalation. When inhaled allergen doesn't make it to the lung, but instead gets trapped in the nose (the most common place allergen gets stuck in the respiratory system), it can trigger allergic inflammatory responses elsewhere in the body, including sending chemicals and inflammatory mediators (signals) via the blood to the lungs and skin.

We want to make sure to control allergic nasal inflammation in children with troublesome or recalcitrant allergic inflammatory asthma. Nasal steroids (the same medications as inhaled steroids, just in different delivery devices) are the best drugs we have for controlling allergic nasal inflammation.

I recommend giving nasal steroids a try (as an additional medication) if you are having any trouble at all controlling allergic inflammatory asthma in your child. In the US, some nasal steroids are now over the counter, and much less expensive than the prescriptions.

Antihistamines

Antihistamines may provide benefit in some children with allergic inflammatory asthma. In most children, they are only of mild value however.

Everyone thinks of antihistamines as the first thing to be taken for allergies, right? Well, I would strongly urge you to think otherwise. Here's a weird thing about antihistamines. In study after study, they don't do diddly to improve chronic allergic diseases like hay fever.

How can that be, you ask? Obviously they work in allergies! And that's right. It is obvious that they work in allergies. Heck, if my eyes start itching, I go straight for the antihistamines, and get relief, fast. Yet the studies say that they don't work.

The answer to this contradictory conundrum is that the studies were designed wrong. It comes from the evidence-based medicine mentality of looking at groups of people to determine average efficacy of drugs. It's a shame, for when it comes to allergies and asthma, we don't *need* to be studying groups. We don't need to rely on group information, because we can study each child as an individual, and pretty easily too. We can see the results of medications in a child pretty quickly in allergic inflammatory asthma. We can do diagnostic empiric trials for asthma and for allergy in each individual child (confounded admittedly by placebo effects, but those can be managed).

I think antihistamines do a little teeny bit, but not much, to help the underlying inflammation in allergic inflammatory asthma. Histamine, after all, is but one of many components of the inflammatory processes in allergic inflammatory asthma. But it happens to be a component that causes itchiness and runny nose: symptoms we definitely notice.

Antihistamines work for us symptomatically (yet don't appear to work for asthma and allergic rhinitis in general in the *studies*) because of how, when, and why we take them. We take antihistamines when symptoms become *bothersome* to us. But here's the thing, there can be a whole lot of inflammation in our nose or lungs before symptoms become bothersome. A little cough or wheeze or booger is not bothersome enough to bother with. But when the eyes start itching, yoweeeee! Treat me now!

Antihistamines knock the tip of the problem away, just enough to make the inflammatory process not bothersome to us, even though the inflammation is cruising along in our airways at nearly full speed. Because the antihistamine knocks away the tip of the iceberg (the bothersome symptoms), a patient will say *"Wow,* these antihistamines work well!" and he will indeed feel better. But the antihistamines don't get to the core of the disease process well, and thus in research studies that look at things other than the symptomatic tip of the iceberg, they don't perform well scientifically.

All that being said, I do prescribe antihistamines often for children who have allergic inflammatory asthma. After all, histamine is often a contributor to asthma, albeit usually a small contributor. I do not prescribe an antihistamine as a standalone medication, that's for sure. Antihistamines should not replace inhaled steroids or montelukast.

Now, some children do really well with antihistamines, because, yep, I'm gonna say it, every child is different, and every situation is different.

Take for example a child who has no cat at home, has allergic inflammatory asthma, is very allergic to cats, and is going to go visit his auntie's house where there are six cats and four-and-a-half kittens. In that setting, I want that child maximally protected against the big allergic assault he is about to undergo, and I will throw the kitchen sink at him in advance of the visit and throughout the visit. Antihistamines are part of that kitchen sink, as are high-dose inhaled steroids, leukotriene modifiers (montelukast usually), albuterol, nasal steroids, and a back-up plan of oral steroids.

Anyhow, antihistamines, especially now that the non-sedating antihistamines are pretty inexpensive, over the counter, and mostly free of side effects, are totally reasonable to try. Give them a go. But not as standalone therapy for asthma.

Other Treatments Possibly Useful in Allergic Inflammatory Asthma

We used to regularly use an inhaled drug called *cromolyn* (brand name: Intal) in children with allergic inflammatory asthma. It is incredibly (completely) safe, and the nebulized version that we can get in the United States is often somewhat cheaper than the current prices of inhaled steroids, although its price seems to bounce around. Cromolyn didn't work in all children, which shouldn't be a surprise to anyone, but it worked in some children. We probably always dosed it too low. Also, we weren't any better back then than we are now at targeting the right drugs to the right causes of asthma. Cromolyn is still out there on the market. Cromolyn is supposed to be used every day (multiple doses a day, like 3 or 4 even) to prevent asthma exacerbations. It is said to take a month to start working.

I often wonder if the reason we stopped using it is because it went off patent and no sales force from a drug company was pushing it on us doctors. There were other drugs more profitable to sell to us, and we doctors paid attention to the sales hype. But I also suspect that cromolyn went through the FDA regulatory process at simply too low a dose, and now the manufacturers and doctors are bureaucratically stuck with it. FDA makes it too expensive to go through that regulatory process again at a more appropriate dose.

It is still debated how cromolyn works. It may stabilize mast cells (remember those cells in the airway and skin and gut that release histamine and a bunch of other inflammatory compounds?). It may work by blocking the acid/heat/capsaicin sensors in the lung. And there are other ways it probably helps in asthma.

Anyhow, I am all for giving it a go. Why not? Cromolyn is harmless, not overly expensive, and may help! It's one of those older drugs that as doctors we should be paying more attention to. As a side note, it often works well to prevent exercise-induced asthma.

There is an old drug called *theophylline* that comes in many forms, swallowed and intravenous. It used to be our main therapy for asthma. It still has a role to play in some children with asthma, but has been thrust aside by newer and safer therapies in general.

I had earlier mentioned *allergy immunotherapy* as a treatment for allergy in general, and many allergists will use careful allergen injections or sublingual drops (under the tongue) to desensitize a child to relevant allergens to which he is allergic. Some allergists will not use these treatments for asthma. Some children with asthma will get sicker with allergy immunotherapy, so this therapy is not without risks. Unlike so many other medications used in asthma, allergy immunotherapy is not something you can do an empiric trial with. If side effects are tolerable and it doesn't make asthma worse, it still takes 3–5 years to desensitize a child to an allergen. It doesn't always work. On the positive side, allergy immunotherapy is the only potentially curative intervention we know of for allergic inflammatory asthma. Definitely this is something to discuss with the allergist who performed the allergy testing on your child, and also with your child's primary doctor.

There are high-tech medications for allergic inflammatory asthma that focus on specific and relevant inflammatory pathways. The most notable of these is *anti-IgE antibodies*. These are antibodies that are injected (once every 2–4 weeks) in a child to bind up the child's IgE antibodies (the allergy antibodies). *Omalizumab* (Xolair) is the name of the anti-IgE antibody preparation, and it is expensive. Very expensive (like $900–$2,200 per dose!). Generally, therefore, insurance companies are going to control its use (or, more aptly put, control whether they will pay for it or not). Remember, you can pay for it yourself and insurance companies can say nothing about that at all. But it costs you a lot of money.

Omalizumab is officially approved for children 12 years old and older, but doctors do not have to obey FDA's approval criteria. They can prescribe the drug to a younger child. But the insurance company will probably refuse to pay for it. Insurance companies use the FDA bureaucracy to avoid having to pay money out.

Omalizumab is generally reserved for the most difficult cases of allergic inflammatory asthma. It is not designed to work in non-allergic forms of asthma, and it doesn't. Most children with allergic inflammatory asthma are readily controlled with environmental modifications (allergen avoidance) and anti-inflammatory medications (steroids and montelukast and maybe a bit more). So when I encounter a child with allergic inflammatory asthma that is not readily controlled with these medications, I wonder if I am missing another diagnosis for her asthma. I go hunting for other diagnoses before I want to try an expensive medication.

Every child is different. Those rare children who have a true failure of function of the steroid receptor in cells, and who have allergic inflammatory asthma, may find omalizumab to be the best thing known to man. And it may be. For children who are allergic to cats, and have a cat in their house, and they have bad asthma, parents should have a sit down with their insurance company and the child and figure out what on earth to do. That $900 to $4,400 per month (the cost of the various regimens of omalizumab) is a heck of a lot of rent to pay to keep a cat. The insurance company may rightfully balk at that. Heck, you might balk at that as a parent too… I know I would. And I love cats. Except that I am so allergic to them that I can't go near them. You can feed a whole orphanage full of children in Africa for a month for $900. That sounds like something your mother would tell you at the dinner table, but even so, it's true. We need to think about these issues. That being said, you have the right to spend *your* money (but not the insurance company's money) however you see fit. It's yours and no one can morally force you not to. If you want to spend your own money to keep the cat, that is totally 100% fine! But really, for the sake of your child, I would encourage you to find the cat a safer home.

Finally, there is a group of children who have what the commonly used guidelines call "severe asthma." That term has become almost a synonym for "asthma that costs a lot of money because of hospitalizations," but to me it is more than that. To me it is "asthma that we have not diagnosed completely, probably because we are missing knowledge about some critical pathologic process that causes asthma that we haven't yet figured out."

And that brings us to a section on *oral steroids*. These are the steroids that are designed to be swallowed, not to be confused with inhaled steroids. This following section is also applicable to injected steroids given at the doctor's office or hospital.

Swallowed oral steroids (most commonly prednisone, prednisolone, or dexamethasone) are our big guns for allergic inflammatory asthma. And they are very powerful and wonderful tools to have in the armamentarium to fight this type of asthma. But they have side effects, and need to be used with caution therefore. I don't want you to have unwarranted fear of them, but nor do I want you to think they can be used willy-nilly.

Generally, oral steroids are used to treat acute exacerbations of allergic inflammatory asthma. Sometimes they are used chronically to treat extremely tough-to-manage allergic asthma, too.

I mentioned this before, but I will say it again. A dose of oral steroids has a whole lot more medication in it than a dose of inhaled steroids does. A typical dose of oral prednisone for a 6-year-old child might be 30 mg (note, dexamethasone is more potent and its doses are smaller). Let's compare this to inhaled steroids. The amount of steroid absorbed into the body from one puff of a steroid inhaler might be 30 *micrograms*, which is 1/1000th the quantity of the prednisone!

I mentioned before that the inhaled steroids are more potent than oral steroids, molecule for molecule, but that means 3–10 times more potent, not 1,000 times more potent. Thus an oral steroid remains a big pump of steroids compared to inhaled — a big solid attack against allergic inflammatory asthma.

The oral steroids go to the body as a whole, instead of primarily to the lungs. Although allergic inflammatory asthma is mostly a lung issue, we recognize increasingly that allergic inflammation tends to affect the body more broadly.

Treating with oral steroids is a wonderful tool. I am so glad we have them available. Oral steroids can melt away allergic inflammation faster than any other tool we have. They start working in a few hours (and have a solid effect in a day) and can get a child healthy when he would otherwise be overwhelmed with allergic inflammation and be sick as a dog. They can keep a child out of the hospital, or get him home faster if he needs to be in the hospital for a bit. Oral steroids are dirt-cheap medications, too—the cheapest of all the asthma medications out there.

How and when are oral steroids used?

There are lots of different ways that doctors use oral steroids in asthma. What I can do here is tell you what I have learned.

My first and key point is that oral steroids are highly effective, but *only in allergic inflammatory asthma.* For other types of asthma, oral steroids may do shockingly little. Those other types of asthma are entirely different diseases, after all, so it is no surprise that a drug will work for one disease well, but not for another.

My second point is that they are used to treat *exacerbations* of allergic inflammatory asthma. In general, the *earlier* oral steroids are started (at the onset of an exacerbation, for example), the *shorter* time they need to be used.

The optimum use of oral steroids requires experience with them and with your child, so that you as a parent can guestimate when to start oral steroids. Your experience as your child's parent, knowing your child's asthma patterns, is the single most important part of the equation when it comes to optimally using oral steroids. Every child is different, so you will need to work with your child's doctor to figure out what is best. But your knowledge from this book will put you in a position to be an excellent collaborator with your child's doctor and with your child, to optimize your child's care.

My third point is basically a summary of the ways I have identified to help a lot of children and parents. As a doctor, I want the parents of my patients to be empowered, and that means they need to be knowledgeable and wise about asthma and asthma treatments. That is the point of this book. Then, after each parent has experience and feels comfortable, I want them to have the armaments against their child's asthma readily available to them. I want them already in their home, without having to wait for a doctor's appointment, or for a called in prescription, or for insurance company approval. Once parents are comfortable, I want them to have oral steroids on hand to treat early an exacerbation of allergic inflammatory asthma.

Not all parents will feel comfortable treating with oral steroids on their own. Some will always want the doctor to see their child before making that decision. For that matter, some doctors will not be comfortable starting oral steroids without seeing the child. In any of these scenarios, the more you know the better off your child will be.

Here's my rule of thumb. If your child with allergic inflammatory asthma has a mild exacerbation of asthma symptoms (from an allergic exposure or from a cold that he has just gotten), then crank up the dosing of *inhaled* steroids way up to 10 puffs or more per day. Also, double (or start) montelukast (if that drug has helped for your child before); treat with bronchodilators every few hours as needed, and see what happens over the next 24 hours. If worsening, then it's time for a dose of oral steroids.

If your child starts with a moderate or bad exacerbation of allergic inflammatory asthma, it is time right away for a dose of oral steroids.

Your doctor can choose the dose, but for prednisone and prednisolone it might be something like 1 milligram of prednisolone per kilogram of body weight, which is about half a milligram per pound. Perhaps 40 mg for a school-age child, 60 mg for a teenager. It's all rough guessing, so struggling over the exact "right" dosage is, well, a waste of time, and quite impossible anyway. Remember that dosing of dexamethasone (a more potent steroid sometimes used in treatment of allergic inflammatory asthma) is much lower than dosing of prednisone.

One dose of oral steroids given early is often all it takes to get ahead of the inflammation. And it is tolerated by most children very well. Sometimes a second dose in a day, or a second or third day of therapy is needed. Doctors often prescribe automatically a five-day course of oral steroids when they think they are needed. That duration of therapy is standard, but it is not focused on *your* child's needs. For any given asthma episode, it may be that your child needs two days of oral steroid, or he might need seven days of oral steroid, or anywhere in between. Five days is just a random number, really. It is best, when possible, to decide what to do as each day passes, based on symptoms primarily, whether another dose or another day of oral steroids makes sense to give. This does not mean that you have to take your child to *see* his doctor each day. Often a phone call is enough, or even just careful instructions/suggestions from your doctor at the beginning as to what to do.

By the middle of the third day of oral steroid treatment, it is common for children to start noticing side effects, and for parents to start noticing the side effects too. (Of course, every child is different.) The most common side effects you and your child will likely experience from oral steroids are:

- Hunger. Lots of hunger.
- Headache. The therapy for this type of headache is eating. Eating is often the only thing that will work. It doesn't have to be much food, but a headache from steroids needs to be fed.
- Behavioral changes. And not for the better, either. Oral steroids can make children misbehave, lose control, get angry, get sad, get irritable, get fussy, get mean. Feeding helps this, for the most part, by the way.
- Sleep disturbance. Can't fall asleep, tossing and turning.

The side effects are no fun.

Children tend to put on weight if they take more than a 5 day course of oral steroids. Some of this is fluid retention weight and goes away just as fast, but some is because they simply have to be eating more. A child with initially normal body weight will return to normal weight soon after stopping the oral steroids. So fear not. The weight gain is more of a concern for children (and parents) who are already overweight. It isn't fair to treat them with medication that makes them need to eat more. Again, early starting of oral steroids leads to shorter courses of them and less side effects, at least in most children. You have to learn your child and her response to oral steroids for yourself.

By the way, oral steroids taste horrible. Yuk... Yuk... Yuk... If your child can swallow pills, use the pills, but they will still be nasty. If your child needs a liquid preparation, well, yuk. Orapred is a branded grape-flavored version of prednisolone and tastes okay but the aftertaste is still nasty. In the United States, it costs about $50, whereas the generic yukkier tasting stuff costs only $10 for a course of therapy. Keep the liquid preparations *cold*. It's a little easier that way. But these meds just taste nasty.

Still, I am glad we have these medications available to us.

CHAPTER 29

Therapy for Other Types of Asthma

Let's move on now to medication therapy for *viral-induced asthma*. Just as a reminder, *viral-induced asthma* is a different entity than *viral-triggered exacerbations of allergic inflammatory asthma*. Please try not to confuse them.

Viral-induced asthma occurs in infants and preschool-age children before they usually can even develop allergies. It results from congenitally small airways, floppy airways, and/or (perhaps most commonly) airways that develop inflammation during colds (such as from overactive acid sensors in the airways). A child with viral-induced asthma gets sick (wheezy, coughing, junky, hard work of breathing) with colds, but between colds the children are usually pretty healthy.

Viral-induced asthma is not as easy to treat as allergic inflammatory asthma usually is.

Mostly, viral-induced asthma is treated symptomatically, which means we do our best to treat the symptoms of the episodes. That involves primarily using bronchodilator medications (usually inhaled albuterol, but sometimes inhaled epinephrine—also known as adrenalin) and keeping fevers down (acetaminophen and ibuprofen). The bronchodilator medication is given by nebulizer most commonly, although it can be given with a metered dose inhaler (MDI) with a facemask. Some children prefer one over the other, and some parents also prefer one over the other. You'll need to decide for yourself. MDIs are quick, but deposition in the airways can be very uncertain in small children. It may take

10 puffs of an MDI to be the equivalent of one nebulizer treatment, but that can vary a lot from child to child. Nebulization takes 10 minutes and deposition in the airway is perhaps a little more certain (especially when given by a mask, but even if given with a corrugated tube device as "blow-by" past the nose and mouth).

Additionally, I recommend treating with acetaminophen for fever (to keep metabolic demands for oxygen lower, and airflow demands less) and also to help keep the edge off the discomfort of having a cold.

As a generality, neither inhaled nor systemic steroids work for viral bronchiolitis, nor do inhaled steroids work particularly well for the viral-induced asthma that the initial bronchiolitis can cause and that can worsen each time a young child gets a cold during the subsequent months and years. Every child is different of course, and it does seem that the inhaled steroids or oral steroids do work for some children with viral-induced asthma. Indeed, I will recommend *trying* them for a while if it seems a child has viral-induced asthma, to see if they work. Inhaled steroids may work in preschoolers who have as yet undiagnosed allergic inflammation, for example. But the inhaled steroids might also work because they are not just anti-inflammatory medications, but also vasoconstrictors (essentially, they decongest). This decongestion effect may be another explanation as to why inhaled steroids are effective in some children with bronchiolitis and viral-induced asthma.

An inhaled steroid (specifically the nebulized budesonide) provides clear help during a viral infection if a child has croup, which can sometimes appear with bronchiolitis or with a viral-induced asthma exacerbation. Croup results from an inflammatory narrowing of the tracheal airway just below the larynx, usually caused by a virus, but sometimes by reflux, allergies, or by unexplained factors. Children with it have very noisy airflow and when they cough it sounds like a bark or like a kazoo (which is also one of the sounds made in tracheomalacia and vocal-cord dysfunction, by the way). Croup is usually a brief illness. Spasmodic croup is often only one night at a time; viral croup usually lasts 3 or 4 nights. A child who croups tends to croup again. Nebulized budesonide helps lots of kids with viral croup, as do swallowed or injected steroids. Controlling fever is important. Usually asthma and croup are not confused, but croup can be confused with aspiration of a foreign body (choking something down into an airway).

It turns out that in clinical studies, leukotriene modifiers (particularly montelukast) have proven effective at reducing symptoms and severity of viral-induced asthma episodes. And that is good news indeed. The leukotriene modifiers can be used once daily for a few years while your child outgrows this type of asthma, or they can be used for a few months each spring and early fall when cold season hits the community.

Will they work to prevent episodes of viral-induced asthma in your child? The only way to know is to try them (and, actually, you may not know for sure one way or the other, because the happy reality is that viral-induced asthma tends to gradually go away as a child grows).

The question often arises: in children with viral-induced asthma, how much does reflux contribute to the worsening and persistence of asthma symptoms? It's a tough question. Nobody knows the answer. I recommend that you try a couple of empiric trials of acid-blockade medication at the onset of viral-induced asthma episodes, and see whether it seems to help in your child. Your assessment will mostly be a gut feeling, but that's okay. Sometimes it is the best information we have.

Therapy for Exercise-Induced Asthma

First, let's clarify the diagnosis of exercise-induced asthma.

Asthma with exercise can occur in the absence of allergies and absence of asthma appearing at any other time. Or exercise can be a triggering event for a child with already-present allergic airway inflammation, or already-present viral inflammation or already-present irritant inflammation (chlorine, smoke, etc.). In all cases, the dehydration of the airway seems to be important at instigating the bronchospasm, which results in coughing and wheezing and shortness of breath during exercise.

But exercise can also cause acid reflux events, and such events can cause wheezing and coughing too. That is an altogether different type of exercise-induced asthma, but it is not easy to tell apart clinically. We often need diagnostic empiric trials to sort it out.

For *children with no other asthma and no allergies* (and if we guess no reflux and no vocal cord syndrome), the treatment options for exercise-induced asthma are many, and *very* effective.

Most commonly, two puffs of albuterol inhaler (with or without a spacer) taken 15 minutes before exercise is an excellent prophylaxis for exercise-induced asthma. The medication will protect against exercise-triggered bronchospasm.

Montelukast taken a few hours before exercise also is effective in many children.

Often just stretching your lungs with deep breathing exercises prior to exercise can help. A warm-up period before exercise often helps.

The best thing to do is to experiment and see what seems to work best.

In *a child who has allergic inflammatory asthma that is triggered by exercise*, the treatment is just a tad bit more complex. In an allergic asthmatic child, exercise triggering asthma symptoms *can* be a sign of ongoing inflammation, or it might just be regular exercise-induced asthma from airway drying. If there are symptoms of asthma unrelated to exercise, then the first step is to better treat inflammation. If inflammation gets under control, that may well be enough to control the exercise symptoms. If there are no symptoms of asthma outside of exercise, then inflammation is probably under pretty good control. Then there are a couple of good options, and they are the same choices that a child without allergic inflammation could consider. One is to use a dose of montelukast in the mornings when exercise is planned. It probably will work fine, and now that the generic is inexpensive, it is a reasonable thing to try. The other option is to use a puff or two of albuterol fifteen minutes before exercise. One of those solutions will probably be all it takes.

I mentioned cromolyn before. So here is a little redundancy from the previous chapter (sorry!). Cromolyn puffers are modestly expensive ($100/canister for 112 puffs) from Canada (I don't think you can get them from US pharmacies anymore); the nebulizer solution is available in the US currently at a variable price ranging from 70 cents to $2 per dose. Cromolyn is considered to be a pretty good drug to prevent exercise-induced asthma, if taken 15–60 minutes before exercise. It is not the cheapest therapy, and probably no better than a couple of puffs of albuterol.

Therapy for Reflux-Induced Asthma

Use of albuterol is a well-recognized risk factor for reflux (because albuterol relaxes the muscle of the valve that is supposed to keep food from coming back up from the stomach). Also, the physiologic disturbance of active asthma (exacerbations) alters the pressures in the belly and the chest, directly increasing reflux.

So when asthma is active, reflux risk increases. If reflux is happening, it can make asthma worse, which can make reflux worse. Round it goes.

But is this an issue with your child? The diagnostic empiric trial is currently the best way to find out. Solid doses of a twice-daily *proton pump inhibitor* (PPI) medication is used to suppress the stomach acid (the most injurious part of reflux, in general). Proton pump inhibitors include the well-known Prilosec (omeprazole) and Nexium (which is pretty much the same drug as Prilosec but has been kept a ton more expensive—although that may change soon). If acid reflux is contributing to your child's asthma, you should see improvement within a couple of weeks, but give the trial a full month at least. If a diagnostic empiric trial confirms (within reason) that acid reflux is contributing to asthma symptoms, then what do you do?

In adults, caffeine, chocolate, and other foods can make reflux worse, and being overweight often worsens reflux too. In children, it's harder to grasp what makes reflux worse and better.

It will be really hard to sort out in your child what foods might be contributing to reflux, if any. And chocolate is just too wonderful a gift to exclude it based on statistics. Although it would be great to change the diet in some minor way to solve reflux in a child, I have rarely seen that happen except in the setting of allergies to infant formulas in babies. But it's certainly a good idea to follow your own instincts in this regard. Just don't fool yourself. Be circumspect and skeptical and as rational as you possibly can be. Obsessing about foods always seems to increase anxiety, and anxiety helps no one.

So, what's left is to (1) control the asthma so that the asthmatic

Many gastroenterologists don't believe reflux causes asthma. But I know unequivocally that it does, in *some* children. I agree with the gastroenterologists that most of the time, reflux is not an issue, but when asthma is flaring, in some children at least, it *becomes* an issue. There is a *ton* of debate about the role of acid reflux in asthma, and it has not been resolved. That's the great thing about dealing with asthma though. You can try the diagnostic empiric trials in *your* child and get pretty good evidence one way or the other that can mostly resolve the debate for *your* child. And all the rest is just academic.

physiology disturbance does not increase reflux, and (2) suppress the acid with ongoing acid-blocking medicines.

High-dose proton pump inhibition is usually not necessary after the diagnostic empiric trial is accomplished. A child's stomach acid can usually be controlled with either lower-dose PPI or with a generally weaker class of acid-suppression drugs called H_2-antagonists. Zantac (ranitidine) and Pepcid (famotidine) are well-known examples of this class. Your doctor can provide guidance as to how to use these, but here are my thoughts.

First, after a full month of PPI at high dose, I do not recommend stopping acid blockade entirely, not right away. Even if the diagnostic empiric trial of high-dose PPI utterly failed to make the asthma symptoms better (which may well happen if reflux is not causing the problem, of course), don't just stop PPI. There is a transient sort of stomach acclimatization to PPIs that is common, and it leads to stomach-acid *excess* when a PPI is stopped suddenly. Instead of stopping them suddenly, I recommend replacing the PPI with Zantac or Pepcid (or their generic equivalents) for 2–3 weeks until the stomach gets used to not having a PPI in the system, and only after that (if the trial was negative) stopping the acid blockade entirely. If the trial was positive, staying on the H_2-antagonist for a prolonged course (often a year or more) is likely sensible.

H_2-antagonists are well tolerated with few side effects. They are not as strong acid suppressors as PPIs are, but are even safer drugs, and very often sufficient to protect a child from acid reflux asthma. But if, after a positive diagnostic empiric trial with the high-dose PPI (confirming acid reflux asthma), the subsequent change over to the H_2-antagonist leads to a recurrence of worse asthma, it may be that your child needs the

PPI long-term. In that case, probably a low dose of PPI will work. You will need to experiment to see what works well for your child. Severe acid reflux–induced asthma may require treatment with both PPI and H$_2$-antagonists given every day, or even more aggressive therapy to control reflux, often under the auspices of a pediatric gastroenterologist.

Now, reflux brings food as well as acid up from the stomach and potentially into the airway. The acid blockade does not stop non-acid reflux. If food is trickling down into the airway and causing asthma problems, that is something that is not readily treatable with medications. Working with your doctor to deal with reflux, or with a wise pediatric gastroenterologist, then becomes more important. It is hard to prove that non-acid reflux is causing asthma. But we can get supportive evidence with radiographic studies and even with bronchoscopic suction of the airways and testing secretions for the presence of food.

Therapy for Irritant-Induced Asthma

Asthma caused by irritants like chlorine gas and cigarette smoke and wood stoves are best treated by avoidance of the exposure, if at all possible. Drug therapies that we have currently available just don't work very well. The best medication we have to offer is symptomatic treatment with bronchodilators.

I have talked about wood stoves already and about cigarettes.

But how about pools? Avoidance of pools with chlorine is no fun at all, and seems unfair to a child. I am working on a drug to help with chlorine- and acid-induced asthma, but it won't be available for a while. So for now, try a couple of puffs of albuterol and a couple of puffs of an inhaled steroid (or a nebulizer of an inhaled steroid) a half an hour or so before going to the pool. This combination may well help your child avoid symptoms caused by the chlorine, at least while he is there swimming. It is possible he may have asthma later that night, and if so, I would symptomatically treat with albuterol for a couple of days.

A cromolyn nebulizer treatment (or a few puffs of cromolyn from an MDI bought from Canada) is also something to try before going to the pool. It might work very well for your child.

Therapy for Vocal Cord Syndrome

This is mostly discussed in the chapter devoted to this illness (chapter 18). But as a quick reminder, the most important thing about vocal cord syndrome is to *know that it exists.* Knowing it exists is the single best way to protect your child from being misdiagnosed with some form of asthma, which will fail to improve with normal asthma therapy. Your awareness of vocal cord syndrome could protect your child from being prescribed chronic oral steroids, and from the chronic side effects that result from oral steroids. Knowing it exists and determining if it seems likely to be happening in your child is the first and most important step to treating it.

Therapy for Asthma in Overweight Children

I mentioned that asthma in overweight children is often more of a challenge to deal with. But regardless of the weight of your child, as always, seek the diagnosis (diagnoses) and direct therapy toward those diagnoses.

I don't really use the concept of obesity in infants and preschool children. They can be healthy chubby kids and end up skinny school-age children. If the parents are both obese, the child is more likely to stay overweight (but that is a statistical thing, not a certainty). If the parents are both trim, a chubby infant rarely stays chubby for more than a couple of years.

But if your child is plump in the school-age years, he or she might stay plump.

If your overweight child is allergic to relevant allergens (stuff that he is actually exposed to), then certainly treat allergic inflammatory asthma.

But consider also that overweight children are more likely to have acid reflux. Perhaps a diagnostic empiric trial directed at that is wise.

Overweight children tend to get out of breath faster because their airways have to support the higher airflow of a higher oxygen demand when they are exerting themselves. Relative narrowing (small or normal airway size with high airflow) can lead to wheezing symptoms. In this case, there is no inflammation to treat, and no bronchospasm to address. Such children wheeze because of laws of physics. It is fine to try bronchodilators to see if they help. If they do, that is because there is a bit of bronchospasm. If they do not, that should not be a huge surprise.

If your overweight child has no allergies, if a diagnostic empiric challenge for acid reflux asthma accomplished nothing, if bronchodilators do nothing, and if there is no other evident diagnosis for his asthma, it may indeed be that relative airway narrowing is the problem. Sure, keep trying medications like cromolyn and montelukast as hopeful shots in the dark, because they might help. But it may be that the best intervention is to get your child in good shape.

Overweight children can get in good shape, even while being or staying overweight. Good shape means that the muscles are well-tuned, appropriately sized, and ready to go during exercise. There can be plenty of well-functioning muscle even in an overweight child. In regard to asthma, the key therapy seems to be *exercise* much more so than *diet*. Regular, fun, solid exercise. My favorite exercise is pressing the buttons that turn off the television and the computer. In and of itself, turning off electric toys and powering down social media devices might not make muscles stronger. But children who aren't staring at screens usually want to be outside, and outside means exercise.

CHAPTER 30

Summary

Asthma is not a diagnosis, but a reason to go seeking a diagnosis. Asthma is a physiologic disturbance that consists of recurrent episodes of reversible airflow limitation in the chest.

Asthma occurs when airways are narrowed and obstructed.

Airways can be narrowed and/or obstructed by bronchospasm, inflammation, accumulation of mucus and other material, kinking of the airways, squeezing from the outside, tumors or foreign bodies on the inside, and other means.

There are common and uncommon diagnoses that lead to these causes of airway narrowing and obstruction.

Your child might have one cause, or more than one cause of his asthma. That means your child might have one or more diagnoses.

Diagnosis of the causes of asthma involves careful consideration of a child's history, physical findings, lung-function testing, a chest x-ray, allergy testing, and how the child responds to various diagnostic empiric trials of medications.

Age is an important factor in what type(s) of asthma your child might have.

The diagnoses that underlie your child's asthma may be

1. Allergic inflammatory asthma
2. Viral-induced asthma
3. Exercise-induced asthma
4. Reflux-induced asthma
5. Bronchomalacia (floppy airways)

6. Congenitally narrow airways
7. Relative narrowing (too much airflow for narrow but otherwise normal airways)
8. Irritant-induced asthma
9. Allergic bronchopulmonary aspergillosis

There are many other disorders that can confound the diagnosis of asthma, such as

1. Vocal cord syndrome
2. Laryngomalacia
3. Chronic lung diseases that lead to recurrent infections, such as cystic fibrosis, antibody deficiencies, or immotile cilia syndrome (ciliary dyskinesia)
4. Obesity
5. Pneumonia

Conscientiously working to identify the diagnosis (or diagnoses) underlying your child's asthma is important.

Each diagnosis for asthma is treated with a different therapy.

Each child may respond differently to the therapies chosen.

Asthma therapy should and can be individualized to your child.

The best therapies for your child may change over time.

Environmental modifications are helpful for allergic inflammatory asthma and for irritant asthma.

The amount of medication needed to be given for your child may change as often as day to day, or week to week. Or it might be able to be maintained at a stable dose over time. Medication doses should be adjusted based on symptoms and lung-function tests, as well as the expectation of exposures to allergens.

Asthma changes over time. Your child changes over time. Be flexible. Be wise. Give thought to your child's asthma on a regular basis.

Work with your doctor and your child closely. Be patient. Ask questions. Seek answers.

And as your child gets older, transition responsibility slowly to your child. In teen years, with loving nagging, your child can probably start taking over her therapies. By the time she is 18 and living on her own, she needs to be making the decisions, increasing or decreasing her medications, etc. (if she still has asthma, that is). Perhaps at that time, buy her a copy of the most recent edition of this book. I hope it will empower her as well as you.

Now, go out, jump in a pile of leaves, swim in a highly chlorinated pool, shake lots of people's infected hands, and buy four cats. And a rat.

Or not.

But please do get control of your child's asthma, so that your child may best enjoy everything that the wonder of life has to offer.

Please visit my website www.childasthmaguide.com for new information, answers to questions, and discussions.

Made in the USA
Middletown, DE
22 March 2019